CROSS THE BRIDGE TO RETIREMENT

KEEPING YOUR FINANCIAL FUTURE STRESS-FREE

BY RANDALL 'DOLPH' JANIS

ISBN: 978-1-7337955-0-0

Edited by: Veronica Janis and MaryLynn Kindberg
          Amy Ashby
Compliance edited by: Red Oak Compliance

Warren
publishing

Published by Warren Publishing
Charlotte, NC
www.warrenpublishing.net
Printed in the United States

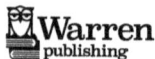

TABLE OF CONTENTS

Acknowledgments.. 5

Introduction 8

Chapter 1
Are you Prepared? 12

Chapter 2
The 4 Cs of Retirement...................................... 25

Chapter 3
The Three Types of Money.................................. 32

Chapter 4
The Truth about Social Security 54

Chapter 5
Safety, Security, and Growth............................... 62

Chapter 6
Health Care Costs in Retirement......................... 81

Chapter 7
Make Taxes Work in Your Favor 92

Chapter 8
Income to Last 111

Chapter 9
Estate Planning 126

Conclusion... 135

About the Author.. 143

Disclosures.. 146

ACKNOWLEDGMENTS

I wish to express my sincere thanks and appreciation to all of those who encouraged, challenged, and cheered me during my developmental years as an athlete, student, and financial professional.

To my mom, Lorrie, and dad, Lawrence, thank you for all your support over the years. Thank you for never missing a game or an opportunity to encourage me, and teaching me that true success comes from giving your best effort, not winning or losing. I love you both for your unselfish participation in my life.

To my best friend and wife, Veronica. I want to thank you for your continued support, patience, and prayers during this often challenging journey in building the company of my dreams. With you and our precious daughter, Samantha, my life is complete. Your beauty outside is the reflection of your beauty inside. I love you with all my heart and soul.

To Veronica Janis and Mary Lynn Kindberg, thank you for your countless hours of careful editing, and for making this book, *Cross the Bridge to Retirement,* as important to you as it is to me and my beliefs.

To Amanda Hogan and Lauren Garvey for all your support and hard work to ensure that the beliefs of Clear Income Strategies Group were not forgotten in this book, as well as your inspiration in naming the book.

To Jeff Conyers for your insight and knowledge regarding Medicare, and for the spirit you bring to the company.

To Warren Publishing and their staff for all their amazing work in making *Cross the Bridge to Retirement* look and be the best it could be.

Lastly, to all my relatives, friends, and clients who in one way or another shared their support either morally, financially, or physically. Thank you.

WHY I WROTE THIS BOOK

As a human race, we are prone to putting things off. We live in a time where procrastination is welcomed. Look at Garfield. He is a prime example of laziness, yet we enjoy his easy-going ways. We all know Garfield disdains any form of exertion or work. He is well-known for saying, "breathing is exercise."

Cross the Bridge to Retirement is a call to action. It is time for us to stand up and start taking control of our lives. I have been a financial professional since 2005, and you can trust me when I say I have seen it all when it comes to finances. I wrote *Cross the Bridge to Retirement* with the goal of assisting people to effectively manage their income and plan for the future. I base my life on the principle that understanding your financial situation *today* is vital to successfully making prudent decisions about *tomorrow.*

This book will help you:
- comprehend retirement concepts
- discover opportunities that could enhance your financial security
- examine the steps you as an individual need to take toward retirement
- understand better your retirement needs.

Nothing about retirement planning is a one-size-fits-all solution. I encourage you to look at the facts from this book and then decide on your own what is best for you. The only way to fully know if these strategies will meet your personal needs is to consult with a local and licensed financial professional who can evaluate your situation.

The best way to handle retirement is to keep it simple. If you engulf yourself in too many unanswered questions and postpone decisions, you could find yourself in a heap of a mess. When it comes to your future, your focus should be on securing your income so you will never outlive your money. No one wants to see their money deplete, or even worse, disappear completely. With a reasonable rate of return and proper planning, your retirement could be a breeze.

The path to retirement is a journey each potential retiree should take as he or she ponders this transition. It is my hope that this book will be the starting point of that journey. *Cross the Bridge to Retirement* is not intended to give investment, legal, or tax advice. It is your job as a consumer to seek out advice from a financial professional. This book also has no intention of giving you the necessary details to choose specific financial products and options. It is wise to first meet face-to-face with a financial professional before making such decisions. Your financial professional should help you ask the right questions, run the numbers, and, if necessary, refer you to additional reliable resources.

I also need to make it clear that nothing is risk-free. Though some financial products and options may come with less risk, I want to be incredibly upfront that everything has a risk of some sort, whether big or small.

That being said, today is the day to start your journey toward retirement—with *comfort* and *confidence.*

Randall 'Dolph' Janis
Financial Professional
(based in North Carolina,
licensed in multiple states)

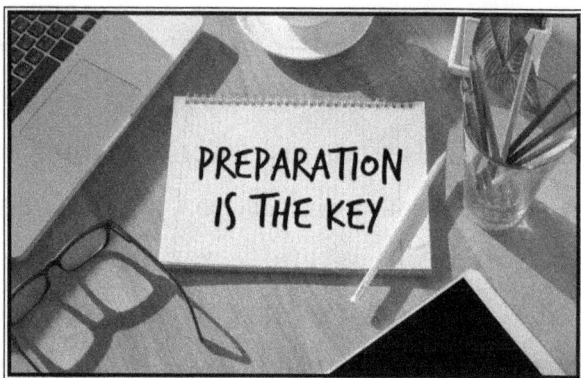

PREPARATION
IS THE KEY

CHAPTER 1
ARE YOU PREPARED?

What would you say if I were to ask about your retirement plans?

Many of us would shrug our shoulders and say, "I'm not old enough for that yet!" In my twenties, I didn't have a care in the world. The last thing I thought about was the day I'd have to retire. I was focused on the here and now, but before I knew it, my twenties were over. My life was moving at such a fast pace, I never stopped to think about tomorrow.

Sadly, financial security in retirement doesn't just happen. Retirement takes high levels of planning and calculation. You cannot simply wake up one day and expect to have it all figured out. The probability of winning the lottery is 1 in 175 million, so unless you are Joan Ginther, the luckiest lottery winner in the world, you will need to financially plan for your future. Keep in mind that *the best way to make money is not to lose money,* as Warren Buffet has often stated.

> *"The best way to make money is not to lose money."*

Most of you feel unprepared for retirement and are worried your nest egg won't be large enough to support you. You are not alone; many Americans feel this way too. A surprising 61 percent of the population is scared to death of outliving their assets. Even worse, 77 percent of people ages forty-four through forty-nine were more scared of outliving their money than they were of dying.[1]

But how can you blame them?

The year 2007 changed many people's points of view on financial security. That year, the US government reported the country's official deficit to be roughly $162 billion. Sadly, the debt was actually closer to $2.5 trillion, about fifteen times worse than officially reported. Four years later, the debt increased to $14.3 trillion, taking into account standing liabilities.

Currently, in order to pay off this kind of debt, each taxpayer would be forced to pay over $100,000. Considering most of us don't have that kind of money, panic has been widespread.

Meanwhile, the national debt has continued to increase at a rate of $2.7 billion per day since September 2013.

And how can we forget the awful stock market crash of 2008 that led to job losses, bankruptcy, and foreclosures? Rest assured there are ways to combat the negative statistics of the market. You *can* have financial confidence in your future.

The average person spends around twenty years in retirement. Imagine going on a trip for a week. First you'll make sure you have everything you'll need for the trip, whether it's clothes, toiletries, or other miscellaneous items. But, if you are like me, you can be halfway to your destination and suddenly realize you forgot your phone charger, or even worse, your phone altogether! Imagine packing for twenty *years*. It's going to take some time and more importantly, it's going to take some planning. You would hate to forget any important details when it comes to your future.

When planning for tomorrow, it is reasonable to expect to live a long life. With better health care and medical advances, people are living much longer. You should never assume you will pass away before you reach the age of retirement. Even worse, you should never assume you will only be in retirement for a short amount of time. It is likely the life expectancy of the most developed countries will continue to advance until it peaks around the age of ninety years old.[2]

You simply cannot afford to be unprepared for your future. Your financial professional can help you take the appropriate steps, outlined below, that could help you find the retirement you are looking for.

Step 1: Decide when you will retire.

Your retirement age will play a huge role toward the amount of money you will need to save before you retire. The age at which you choose to retire can determine how much you can expect from a company pension plan, as well as Social Security benefits. The more income you receive from such plans, the less money you will need to save personally. Any income you receive from pensions, Social Security, or retirement accounts is all a part of the money you will use in your later years. Your retirement age will help determine what accounts are best suited for you. Many accounts have age requirements, surrender periods, and withdrawal provisions, so be cognizant of this as you make your decision.

Step 2: Be open about your vision for retirement.

When talking to your financial professional, everything you would like to do post-retirement needs to be considered. We all have different goals in life, and it is important to understand what these goals may be. Perhaps you have been dying to visit Europe. Or, maybe you want to build a lake house or to just live comfortably and leave an ample inheritance for your loved ones. The clearer your vision, the more likely you are to accomplish those goals. For example, would you like to visit Europe once or more than once? For ten days or for twenty? Alone or with family? And how about that house on the lake? Would it be a cottage or a five-bedroom house? In North Carolina, Florida, or Maine? Every decision has a big impact on those goals.

Ask yourself honestly, "What do I really want to do in retirement?" It is, after all, the last third of your life; how do you want to live it?

Your financial professional can provide options to help you achieve these goals. This way you will have enough money to live today, with the potential growth to enjoy tomorrow, an income stream that you cannot outlive, and, if important to you, a financial legacy to leave your loved ones.

Step 3: Set a budget for retirement.

A budget ensures you have enough money to pay off debt and provide income in the future. Determining your net worth, which is the total value of your assets minus the value of your debt, is a great way to start planning for your retirement.

Don't be disconcerted if your assets are not worth more than your debts. Even if you find your net worth to be negative (as many people do), start there to figure out what you can do to make it positive. Your future depends on the ability of your money to outlive you, not the other way around.

Step 4: Save money in order to provide for future expenses.

Saving money is key; even putting a small amount of money away each month can end up providing a great return.

Imagine if you had been saving your weekly allowance of fifteen dollars since you were a child. After fifteen years you would have saved about $12,000. If you had invested it at a 6 percent return, you would have over $20,000. Many of you are now wishing you could start over, but sadly, none of us are like the movie character Benjamin Button, who aged in reverse. As your grandfather always says, "I'm not gettin' any younger," and, like your grandfather, neither are you.

It is never too late to start saving. Devise a savings plan, then set achievable goals and stick to them. Your saved money will eventually be money you depend on to generate either interest or dividends in your later years. Putting this saved money to work for you now is one of the best ways to improve your chances of a bright financial future.

Again, your saved money, or core capital, should be designed to outlive you, not the other way around. This is key to preparing for retirement. Of course we would like our bank accounts to hit zero the day we pass, but this is not realistic. No one knows how long they will live.

"Don't take my word for it. Let the numbers speak for themselves."

Your financial professional can make sure your core capital earns the highest possible rates with appropriate safety measures. You should always make sure this core capital is protected. It feels good to see your money increase, but it's even better to know it will never decrease. That way, if you live a long life, you are fully protected.

To determine how you can better save for the future, be objective and dig in. As an experienced financial professional, one of my favorite things to say to people is: "Don't take my word for it. Let the numbers speak for themselves."

I encourage you to consistently review and, if necessary, rebalance[3] your financial portfolio. Periodically, you should be checking to make sure the mix of investments and accounts you have is balanced. When you do, you will be surprised to see the potential of your accounts.

You are now ready to buckle down and start thinking seriously about your future. To continue down the path with comfort and confidence, there are a few more things of which to be aware and to consider.

Here is an article I wrote for *fortune.com* in 2015, which I believe is helpful as you begin to plan for retirement.

Featured on *fortune.com*
Article by: Dolph Janis
Published: September 2015

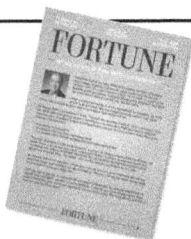

Are You Guessing or Planning for Your Retirement?

Milestones define our lives. Whether it's making the team, graduating from college, or getting that first job, goals are set and dreams are realized. When you reach retirement age, it is important to ensure your financial goals are realistic. Everyone should enjoy retirement. But, there are many factors that can tarnish your Golden Years.

When you are thinking about all the preparations for retirement, i.e. when, where, how, and such, does the thought of safety come to your mind? When I talk with clients, they often worry whether their money will last.

As Warren Buffet has said many times, "The best way to make money is not to lose money." You can accomplish that goal by properly planning for your retirement. First, you need to meet and interview (yes, interview) multiple financial advisors until you find the one who meets these three important requirements:

- Your advisor is trustworthy
- Your advisor has your best interest at heart
- Your advisor offers multiple strategies for your retirement income

Continued on next page

The third requirement is the most important. If a financial advisor only provides one strategy, run away. There is no perfect option that covers every retiree, therefore financial advisors should offer more than one route to retirement. When you find your advisor, test them and let them know about your financial fears. You earned your money, now you need make sure it lasts.

In the past, retirement depended on how much money you had. Now, Americans are working and living longer, but expenses are also increasing. Discover your income value, so you know what to expect out of your retirement.

Let's say at age fifty-five, you have $500K put away for retirement. You are planning to retire at age sixty-two, and need $40K per year to live comfortably. Therefore, you have roughly seven more years to meet this goal. With clear objectives, you can make a plan that is specifically tailored to help you achieve those goals.

In a similar scenario, you hope to receive $50K a year in income, but a market correction causes your savings to drop from $500K to $350K. By not planning for market corrections, you have lost part of your retirement income. This oversight means you might have to rethink your retirement lifestyle.

Certain accounts can provide income riders that will tell you the amount of income you will have seven years later. This way you know exactly what to expect and how to plan for your retirement. To prevent losing part of your retirement nest egg, plan for the retirement you want.

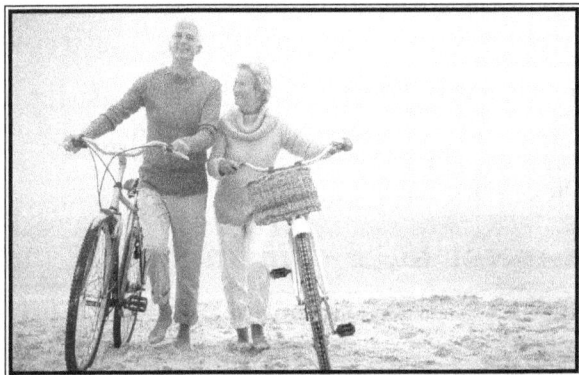

CHAPTER 2

THE 4 Cs OF RETIREMENT

One way to safely cross the bridge to retirement is by looking at the 4 Cs of successful retirement income strategies.[4]

This simple and helpful framework provides an uncomplicated process to help you ask questions and work through the complexities of retirement planning.

Retirement today looks very different than it did generations ago. The financial world is changing and so must our approaches to it. In order to enjoy the retirement you envision, you must first consider the transition—plus the years to follow.

The 4 Cs framework is progressive, and it is meant to be done in a linear order. The 4 Cs discussed below are: **Clarity**, **Comfort**, **Cost of Living**, and **Certainty**. They will help you to think through your needs, wants, concerns, and attitudes toward retirement in a specific and systematic manner. If you are like most Americans, you may be concerned about having enough for your future.

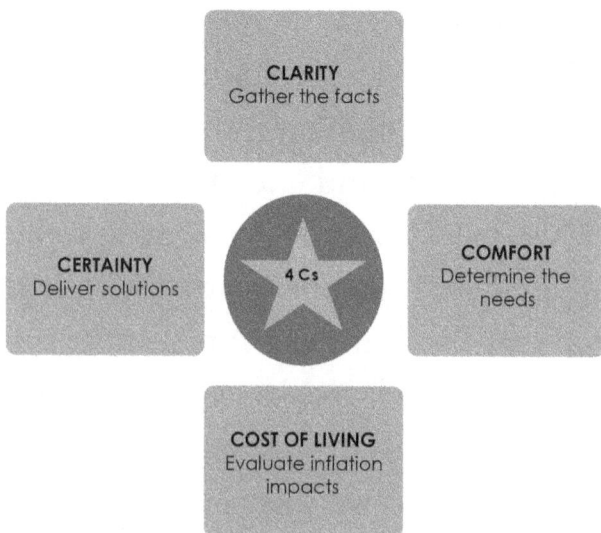

CLARITY
Gather the facts

CERTAINTY
Deliver solutions

4 Cs

COMFORT
Determine the needs

COST OF LIVING
Evaluate inflation impacts

Clarity

Look at the realities of today and then address the following basic questions about tomorrow:

- How much income do you need in retirement?
- How many years might you live in retirement?
- What sources of guaranteed income do you already have?
- What is your "risk tolerance"?
- Do you plan to leave anything to your heirs or charities?

Your financial professional should help you through these questions to calculate how much income you will need. This is important in order to clarify your retirement scenario.

Even though this figure can vary widely from person to person, most estimates indicate you will need at least 70 to 80 percent of your current income. This lays a strong foundation for your retirement savings. Predicting a long life is essential to ensure you have income to last, since many Americans today could spend twenty or more years in retirement.

It is also necessary to clarify what your extra sources of income are in retirement. Sources of income like Social Security, savings accounts, IRAs, 401(k)s, and annuities provide you with supplemental income in your later years.

If you do not have other sources of income, you should still know your risk tolerance. Risk tolerance is an important component in investing. It refers to the degree of variability in investment returns that an individual is willing to withstand. It is wise to have a realistic understanding of your willingness to see large swings in the value of your investments. This can help determine what financial options are more suitable for you. Certain market financial products carry high risk while others offer lower interest rates but greater safety.

Comfort

Decide what kind of lifestyle you want to enjoy for what could be multiple decades of retirement living. When it comes to retirement planning, most of us have one goal in mind: that our money will be there for us to maintain our current lifestyle. A financial professional can help you re-frame your retirement strategies so you can afford the lifestyle you want.

Cost of Living

Evaluate the impact of inflation on retirement savings. Inflation is beyond anyone's control, but you can prepare by tracking your spending patterns and by estimating the price increases. For example, the one hundred dollars you now spend on groceries could end up buying you half as many groceries in twenty years if the current rate of inflation remains steady.

Inflation can drastically affect your savings. It can also increase your health care costs. It is true health care costs have risen faster than the average annual income. In fact, annual family premiums rose 5 percent to average $19,616 in 2018.[5]

Your financial professional should suggest retirement strategies that take into account these serious consequences of inflation.

Average Annual Premium Change from 2000–2018

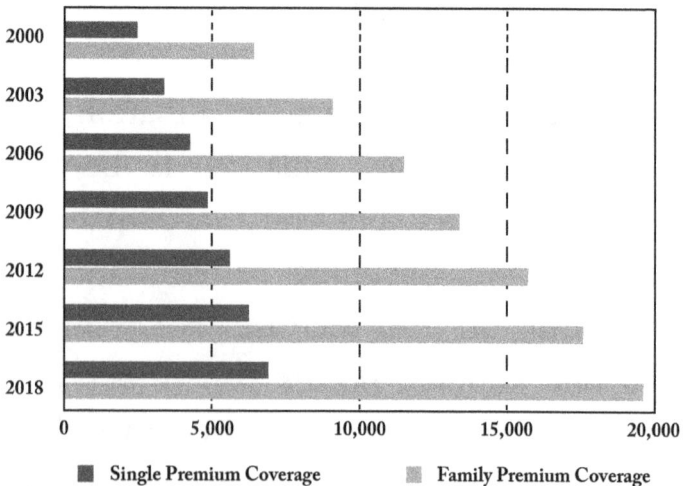

Source: Kaiser/HRET Survey of Employer-Sponsored Health Benefits

https://www.kff.org/interactive/premiums-and-worker-contributions-among-workers-covered-by-employer-sponsored-coverage-1999-2018/#/?compare=true&coverageGroupComp=family&startYear=2000

Certainty

Once you accept your financial reality, define the lifestyle you want to maintain, and factor in the inevitable effects of inflation, you can live with the certainty that your retirement goals and strategies are realistic and manageable.

The truth about your financial scenario today and a comparison with what tomorrow could look like can give you the certainty that will set you free. A financial professional should offer you multiple strategies designed to meet your long-term retirement needs. Then, by utilizing proper income sources, you can enjoy the certainty of having enough income to last, no matter how long you live.

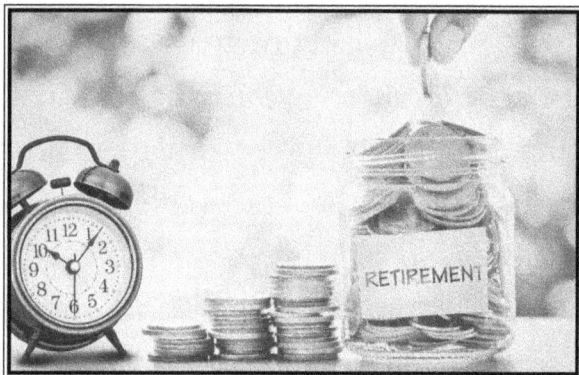

CHAPTER 3

THE THREE TYPES OF MONEY

As your comfortable journey toward retirement continues, there are three types of money to consider before you can reach that well-deserved stage: "today money," "tomorrow money," and "never money." As you will see, they are very different and are to be used in very different ways.

Today Money

I realize a lot of your "today money" is used to pay bills and buy everyday necessities. However, it would be wise to put some today money into short-term investments that will help you save toward retirement. Short-term investments include **CDs, money markets,** and **fixed annuities.** The advantage of these investment options is their short "surrender" period that can increase the money in your savings account in just a short amount of time.

If you spend your today money on a new television or a slick new speedboat, you won't have any money left for these all-important short-term expenses. The general rule of thumb is to always have enough liquid money available. No, I do not mean money in the form of H_2O. Liquid money means money you have readily available. If your yearly expenses are $75,000, you should have $75,000 in savings toward retirement.

Have you been investing your today money wisely or spending every last penny? Short-term investments can be a great opportunity and can come in many different forms. Discuss with your financial professional which short-term investment option can best work for you. The last thing you want is for your today money to be here today and totally gone tomorrow. I have listed for you some alternatives for short-term investments:

CDs

CDs (Certificates of Deposit) are a commonly known and commonly owned type of short-term investment. They are a type of savings account with a fixed interest rate and fixed date of withdrawal. One of the biggest advantages of investing in a CD is that the FDIC insures them up to $250,000. CD rates fluctuate according to the Federal Reserve and can be purchased with varying term lengths. Generally speaking, CDs with longer-term maturity will offer higher rates of return. CD investments offer three different payment options for you to receive your interest: check, direct deposit, or capitalized payments that are automatically reinvested back into the CD.

Money Markets

Money markets also cater to short-term investment needs. Opening a money market account is as easy as opening a savings account. The only criteria for the account is having a minimum balance that remains untouched for a certain amount of time.

Money market accounts also offer a higher interest rate than if you were to simply leave your money in a savings account. Money market accounts yield a percentage of return based on interest rates and the amount of money you hold in your account. Since 2013, money market accounts held a return rate of 0.42 percent or higher, depending on the type of investment.

Although they may not have a high return, money market accounts are a very low-risk investment option. Previously, the US government did not insure the majority of money market funds, but today, most are. This means even if your bank or credit union goes out of business, your money will still be readily available to you.

Fixed Annuities[6]

Fixed annuities offer many advantages when looking for other ways to invest your today money. For one, fixed annuities have tax-deferred growth, which means the interest earned is not taxed until it is touched. Your funds grow without any tax deductions. Another benefit of tax-deferred annuities is that at any time, you can change from a savings or accumulation vehicle to an income vehicle. When I say "vehicle," I do not mean the car you drive. Vehicle can be translated to different types of programs or account options.

Fixed Annuities are one of the safest guaranteed options available. Baseball legend Babe Ruth is one who invested 100 percent of his funds into annuities. His famous quote still resonates today: "I may take risks in life, but I will never risk my money. I use annuities and I never have to worry about my money." He is absolutely right. Annuities provide safety, security, and protection from the unknown. What is best, annuities can provide an income that cannot be outlived.

Luckily there are many different annuity options. Some are more suitable for today and others are more suitable for tomorrow, depending on term length. Interest rates on annuities are usually higher than bank CDs or other fully guaranteed products. Additionally, unlike bank CDs, annuities give you access to your funds even while they earn interest. Generally, Fixed Annuities have no contract fees or sales commissions that are payable by the owner of the annuity. Due to the many added benefits, features, and accessibility, annuities are rapidly becoming one of the most popular options for retirement planning.

Tomorrow Money

Planning for retirement is about saving money in such a way that you can live confidently in the future. (Why sit on the floor when you could be resting easy on a fancy recliner?)

It is always good to be prepared for tomorrow. Sadly, we enjoy the sense of security in the moment and often forget about what the future may hold. We want to be protected here and now, but it is necessary for us to look beyond the present. Preparing for tomorrow can look like a lot of different things, but hopefully it includes a means of saving and protecting your money.

"Tomorrow money" is just that—for tomorrow. It is money you plan on leaving untouched until you retire. In contrast to today money, tomorrow money is what you invest over a prolonged period of time.

Some investment options geared toward saving for tomorrow without risk include: **life insurance policies** and **retirement guarantees.** The advantage of these investment options is their higher interest rates, since they require you to maintain the accounts for longer periods of time. The following strategies are appropriate for investing for tomorrow:

Life Insurance Policies

There are three different ways to handle a life insurance policy: the right way, the wrong way, and the sad way. The right way would be opening the policy and following all of the policy recommendations and requirements. The wrong way would be just like what would have happened in elementary school if your teacher had asked you to complete a homework assignment the night before; hopefully you wouldn't have come in empty-handed the next day. But, if you had, then you would have known the penalty: a bad grade and maybe even a phone call home to your parents. Though the insurance company will certainly not tattle on you to your family, if you do not follow the policy requirements, you will still face penalties. The sad way to handle a life insurance policy is by passing away. Though it is sad, the money from the policy is passed down to your beneficiaries and can provide for them in an incredible way.

Why is it beneficial to own a life insurance policy? What are the different types of life insurance policies?

Life insurance policies are beneficial because they provide different combinations of death benefit protection and accumulation potential. Generally, the more flexible your premium payments are, the greater your chances for tax-deferred cash value accumulation. Life insurance policies are either "term policies" or "permanent policies."

Types of Life Insurance

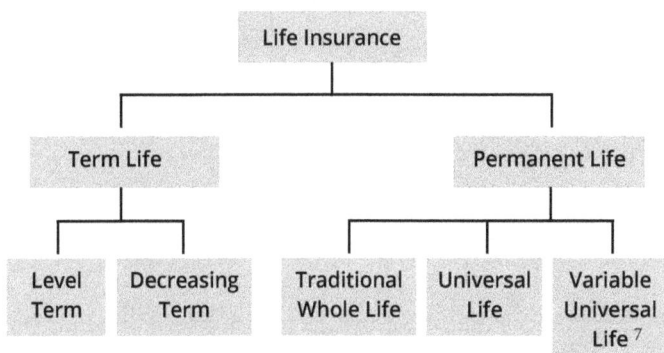

```
                    Life Insurance
            ┌──────────────┴──────────────┐
        Term Life                    Permanent Life
       ┌────┴────┐          ┌─────────────┼─────────────┐
     Level   Decreasing   Traditional  Universal   Variable
     Term      Term       Whole Life      Life      Universal
                                                     Life [7]
```

Term life insurance provides coverage for a specified period of time, after which the coverage stops and the policy terminates. Though they do offer predictable premium payments, term policies are meant to serve as a death benefit only.

Permanent life insurance can be broken down into **whole life insurance, universal life insurance,** and **fixed index universal life (FIUL) insurance.**

Whole life insurance offers the predictability of what are known as level premium payments. These are payments that never increase and can provide coverage for your entire life. Whole life insurance policies also have cash value, which you can access through loans and withdrawals from your policy.

Universal life insurance can provide coverage for your entire lifetime. This product offers flexibility to pay your premiums at any time and in any amount as long as the policy expenses and cost of coverage are met. Universal life policies also have cash value that can accumulate at a fixed interest rate, which you may access through policy loans and withdrawals.

Fixed index universal life (FIUL) insurance[8] also provides death benefit protection. The only difference is that it accumulates cash value based on positive changes of an external index. As a result, this gives it greater accumulation potential than traditional universal life insurance. There is also a built-in annual floor that ensures your cash value will not decrease due to market volatility. The money from this product is never directly invested in the market.

Retirement Guarantees

Guaranteed retirement income can help ensure your money for tomorrow. In order to build a stable foundation for guaranteed income, you can invest in **annuities, pensions,** and **longevity insurance.**

Annuities can be either "immediate," "fixed," or "variable." They are a great way to create guaranteed income. When you purchase an immediate annuity, you deposit a lump sum of money into an account for a specified amount of time. As the name suggests, these annuities start paying out right away. A variable annuity[9] is more futuristic in that you deposit funds today and the annuity company watches the account for you. As that amount increases with interest from year to year, your account value grows and you lock in to a higher "base income."

Both immediate and variable annuities come in many shapes and sizes. As I said previously, fixed annuities are a great way to invest today money, but because there are so many different forms of annuities, they can also be a good way to invest tomorrow money. Fixed index annuities[10] are similar to variable annuities in that they have similar variable rates of return. Despite this fact, there is one major difference: you cannot lose money in a fixed index annuity. Performance is based on a specific index and not invested into the market. With a fixed index annuity, the value of your account can only go up. Your financial professional should help you sort out the different kinds of annuities in order to find what option is best for you.

Pensions, as you know, are contracts for a fixed sum to be paid regularly to a person once they have reached the age of retirement. A pension set up by an employer is called an *occupational* or *employer pension*. The money used to fund this type of account is usually generated by both the employer and the employee. Your payout typically depends on your salary and how long you have worked for a company. Once you retire, you can receive this money either in one lump sum, or in monthly payments from an annuity. With pension plans, I do use "guaranteed" loosely for the simple fact that it is possible for such plans to get into a financial mess—pensions can be cut, defaulted, or even disappear. In order to prevent this from happening to you, there are forms of government insurance programs from an organization called the Pension Benefit Guarantee Corporation that are set to protect pension benefits.

Longevity insurance is a deferred immediate annuity that will guarantee you a minimum amount of income, starting at a specific age. People usually choose longevity insurance to provide them with mental security so they can spend their assets on fun and/or travel during retirement. This type of insurance also has a guaranteed floor of income that will be available if you are to live longer than expected.

Many of us do not expect to live well into our 90s, but the truth is, people are living longer and longer each year. Living longer than you had expected could strain your financial resources and leave you high and dry. With this form of guaranteed income, there is no need for you to worry about what you will do financially if you end up living a long time.

Never Money

"Never money" is just that—money you will never personally touch. This money is for you to hand down to loved ones, use for family debt, or donate to charity.[11] There are many ways to preserve and protect this type of money instead of hiding it in your freezer or stuffing it under your mattress!

First and foremost, you need to make sure that even though you are tempted to touch this money, you stick to your goals of preserving a large sum until after you have passed. In this way you can be assured you will not outlive your money, and you have something to pass to your heirs.

The worst thing you can do is wake up one day, pull money out of your account, and go buy something on a pure whim. Withdrawing money could cause you to lose principal, interest, and tax benefits. Even worse, withdrawing money from accounts before their surrender period could leave you paying withdrawal penalties. Money you planned to never touch could get depleted to almost nothing if you are not careful and disciplined.

"Spending your 'never money' is a deadly retirement savings sin."

Investment options to preserve and protect never money include: **life insurances policies** and **different types of annuities designed for beneficiaries (a.k.a. legacy annuities).**

Life Insurance Policies

Life insurance can be the ultimate gift to your heirs. It can provide the reassurance your loved ones will be protected should the unexpected occur. As you know, the main reason for buying life insurance is to provide a death benefit for your loved ones; however, it can also help supplement the cost of your children's or grandchildren's education.

Supplementing college funding is the most widely used option. For example, if you gift premiums to your son or daughter, they can purchase a life insurance policy on their own lives and name their children as beneficiaries to protect their kids in the event of your son's or daughter's premature death. Also, if you open a life insurance policy on yourself, and add your grandchildren as beneficiaries, in the event of your death, your grandchildren will receive the tax-free death benefit, which can be used to help fund their college education.

Additionally, the policy's cash value has the potential to accumulate tax-deferred. The available cash value can be accessed through loans or withdrawals. Using these funds to help your grandchildren through college comes with no complex eligibility requirements, no qualified education costs, and no income limits to consider.

Also, a policy loan or withdrawal will generally not affect your grandchild's eligibility to receive other forms of financial aid. With tuition rising faster than the rate of inflation, funding a college education is a bigger than ever expense for most families.

It is not important how much money you have, but how much income you receive.

To simplify the three types of money, here is an article I wrote for *money.com* in 2015 about today, tomorrow, and never money.

Featured on *money.com*
Article by: Dolph Janis
Published: April 2015

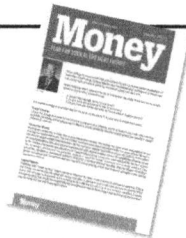

Plan for your retirement future

When talking to so many potential and current clients, a common theme among them is the fear of not having a proper plan for their retirement and running out of money, and not having a proper plan in place arises over and over.

When thinking about different forms of retirement planning, there are three simple questions the investor is smart to ask:

- Do you have enough money to use today?
- Do you have enough money to live on tomorrow?
- Do you have any money put away as "never money" (legacy money)?

It is a great strategy to start planning for the three topics above. It is quite easy to break them down.

Today's Money

This is the money you need to live on today to support your lifestyle, and it includes home costs and everyday activities. Generally, this money is kept in banks or credit unions for the sake of easy access, but usually, it doesn't yield much interest.

Tomorrow Money

Moving into tomorrow money. This is your retirement money: The money you have saved and planned to use during your retirement years. The use of fixed and fixed index annuities are great for this stage of your life as you can receive a guaranteed lifetime income for you and your spouse that neither of you can outlive. It also offers principal protection. This allows you to earn interest with market indexes without the possibility of losing money in the market.

Continued on next page

The money you should put into these products is the money you want watched for the rest of your life. As always, guaranteed and principal protection apply to certain insurance and annuity products (not securities, variable, or investment advisory products) including optional benefits, and are subject to product terms, exclusions, and limitations and the insurer's claims-paying ability and financial strength of the issuing insurance company.

Legacy Money

Finishing with "never money." Legacy money is forgotten by many when it comes to retirement planning. This is the money you never plan on using; the money you plan on giving to your loved ones, heirs, or to charity. What makes this strategy so important is if something in your life were to arise (such as a medical condition, a family emergency, etc.), this would be considered your emergency money. In short, legacy money is the money you don't plan on using but feel safe knowing is there.

There is no such thing as a perfect plan for your retirement. But having the systems in place to help protect your retirement is a step in the right direction. It doesn't matter how much money you have, but more importantly, how much lifetime income you have that continues to produce money.

Where to put and protect your money is always a hard decision, and many people don't like insurance companies.

I am going to put this thought in your head, not just for you, but also for your friends and colleagues.

- If you own a car—do you have car insurance?
- If you own a home—do you have home owner's insurance?
- If you are married or have children—do you have life insurance?
- Do you have health insurance?

I think it is safe to say that your car, your home, your family, and your personal wellbeing are the four most important parts of your life.

Well, if you were going to have these protected with an insurance company, then why, may I ask, why would you not want to protect your retirement and future with one too?

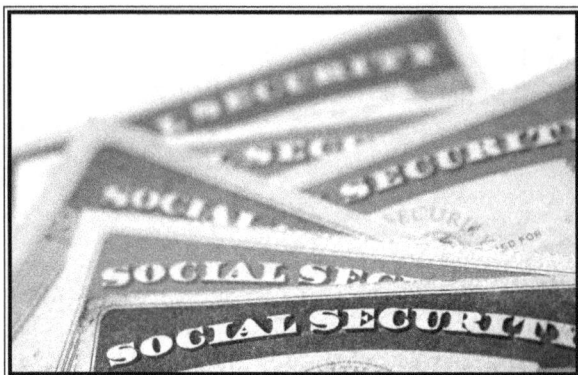

CHAPTER 4

THE TRUTH ABOUT SOCIAL SECURITY[12]

As people near retirement, questions always pop up about Social Security. Can I depend on it to help supplement my retirement? What should I expect from my Social Security benefits? Are all the negative things I've been hearing about it true?

In 1935, if you were sixty-five or older, you received Social Security payouts that would last twelve to fifteen years. That means you would essentially be covered until you were about seventy-eight. The only problem with this today is that people are living well past the age of eighty-five. Social Security was never built to sustain a long retirement. The average life expectancy has drastically changed since 1935, and continues to change.[13]

Hopefully, you are not one of the many depending on Social Security alone to fund your retirement. The cold-hard truth is that Social Security is failing even faster than anyone imagined. Over the long haul, Social Security has promised trillions of dollars more in benefits than the nation could ever pay. Because programs like Social Security are funded through payroll taxes, money will continue to be there as long as workers are readily available. However, our country now has a larger amount of baby boomers retiring and a smaller number of workers contributing to the fund.

Analysts believe the program will eventually no longer be able to pay out the full benefits that were promised. Without changes, Social Security in 2033 will be able to pay only seventy-five cents for each dollar of scheduled benefits. This may have a negative impact on your retirement.

Although Social Security is by far the largest source of income for most elderly Americans, it was never intended to be the only source of retirement income. If you want to prepare for the unexpected and take control of your future, don't put all your eggs into the basket of Social Security.

Although we've established that Social Security will not be able to fully fund your retirement, you will still need to decide when you want to start drawing out your benefits. You may be able to start drawing Social Security benefits as early as sixty-two years old. However, if you do wait until the full retirement age of sixty-six, you'll be eligible for the maximum amount of payouts. Though the amount may be small, it is still in fact your money.

Changes in benefits received according to Full Retirement Age
(based on $1,500 in monthly benefits)

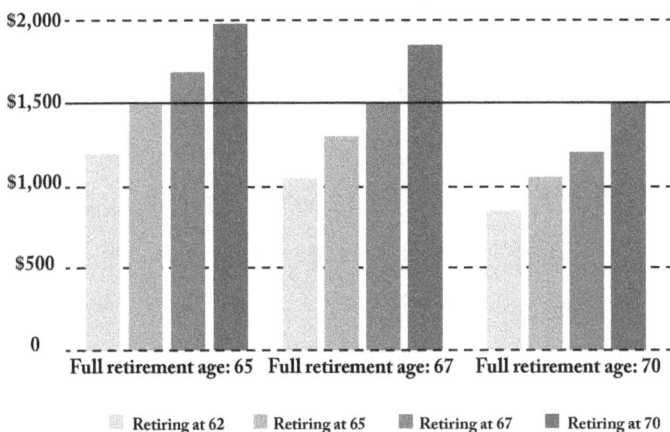

Information based on Social Security Administration

https://www.ssa.gov/planners/retire/ageincrease.html, and https://www.cbpp.org/research/social-security/social-security-benefits-are-modest#retirementAge

The longer you wait to start taking your Social Security benefits, the larger your monthly payment will be. If you have other sources of retirement income available to you, it may be wise to delay taking Social Security payouts. A financial professional can help you determine whether delaying payments is a good strategy in your situation.

Benefits are estimated according to "credits" you have earned.[14] Credits come from the amount of time you have been working. In 2019, you earn one credit for each $1,360 of income. The maximum you can earn is four credits per year. Most people need at least forty credits earned over their lifetime in order to receive retirement benefits.

If you work while taking Social Security, there are limitations.[15] If you are under your full retirement age, you give up $1 in benefits for every $2 you earn over the annual limit. For 2019 that limit is $17,640. However, if you are within the year of reaching the appropriate age of retirement, you only give up $1 in benefits for every $3 you earn over $46,920. Once you reach your full retirement age, your benefits will no longer be reduced.

If you were to become disabled before retirement age, you could receive disability benefits after six months. However, you must have had six to twenty credits earned at least three to ten years before you were disabled, and a physical or mental impairment preventing you from working for at least a year.[16]

If you are applying for Social Security as a couple, you may claim either your own benefit or a derivative of your spouse's. In this case, you are able to take the higher benefit. When it comes to Social Security benefits for spouses, the determining factors are the length of marriage, work history, and the ages of both spouses.

Each spouse needs roughly ten years of work history to qualify for individual benefits. The spouse with the stronger work history must apply for Social Security retirement benefits in order for the other spouse to collect.

Your financial professional can help you obtain your Social Security statement, review your current benefits, and show you how these benefits can fit into your overall retirement income strategy. If you find out you have a gap in income, you will need to plan accordingly and make informed decisions.

So, if you can't depend solely on Social Security, then what else is there? You may also have money saved, but how can you be sure it is enough? You probably have looked into investing in a 401(k) or an IRA, but how can you be sure if they're right for you? Will investments like these really provide the dependability you need in retirement? Well, be assured you have plenty of safe options that your financial professional can offer you. Your financial professional should also be able to provide you with various software programs that can help you plan your Social Security payouts and better understand how much you should expect each year.

Ironically, many people do not like annuities, or even hearing the word. In reality, Social Security is an annuity. There are only three sources of guaranteed lifetime income: Social Security, income annuities, and pensions. Again, money is nice, but lifetime income will protect you from the fear of outliving your money.

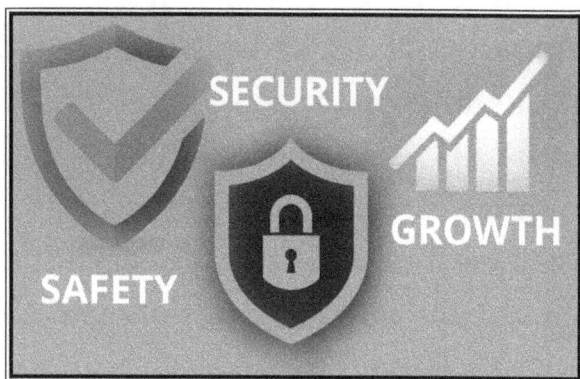

CHAPTER 5

SAFETY, SECURITY, AND GROWTH

We all tend to think like my client Judy did not long ago: she thought putting money into a savings account at the bank was the safest way to guarantee her retirement income. And, of course, Mr. Bankman was more than happy to take Judy's money, but sadly banks are not just thinking about you.

The interest you are accumulating from having your money in the bank is but a fraction of what Mr. Bankman is making off of you. You see, Mr. Bankman takes every $1 you deposit, pays you a measly 1 percent in annual interest, and then turns around and creates $5 through fractional reserve banking, which allows banks to lend out the vast majority of their deposits on hand.

As you can see, the benefits are more for the banker than for yourself. If Mr. Bankman were to lend out $5 at 6 percent interest for every $1 he pays out at 1 percent interest to you, he would be making a profit of 3,000 percent! Also, take into account that the interest you are actually accumulating is heavily taxed, and then depleted by inflation.

Some people ask, "How about Wall Street?" When you invest your money into Wall Street, you are putting yourself at risk. The problem with the stock market is that investors are spurred by three characteristics: emotion, greed, and risk taking. These three together combine to make for really poor financial success. People just like you have found their accounts wiped clean by margin calls and losses.[17]

This is a dangerous situation if you are depending on invested money to carry you through retirement.

If the market goes up 10 percent and then down 10 percent, are you even?

The answer is NO, you will always have that 1 percent loss.

Example:
$100,000 + $10,000 (from 10% up) = $110,000
Then,
$110,000 - $11,000 (from 10% down) = **$99,000**

So, where does this leave you as a current or future retiree? What can protect you against market losses and give you a better return than just squirreling away your money in a savings account? The answer: Fixed Annuities.

In Chapter 3, annuities were briefly mentioned, but I would like to take the opportunity to describe them here in greater detail. As previously stated, an annuity can be an important part of a solid retirement plan and can assure some of your income lasts as long as you do.

What actually *is* an annuity? An annuity is an agreement between you and an insurance company. You give money to an insurance company and, in return, they give you a guarantee. With some annuities, that means guaranteed income for a set period of time or for the rest of your life. Annuities are similar to Social Security or pension plans that you fund yourself.

Annuities can do other things as well. They can grow money that is tax-deferred and is guarded against market risk. They can also be customized with riders that can be added at an additional cost. Some riders include guaranteed lifetime income and the potential for increasing income in retirement to protect against inflation.

Let's take a look at different types of annuities that are designed to do different things.

Fixed Annuities

A fixed annuity is right for you if you want protection from market loss and the predictability of knowing exactly how much interest and income you will receive. Fixed annuities earn steady or fixed interest for a specified period of time and they protect your money from the drama of the stock market.

Fixed annuities historically pay higher interest rates than bank CDs, plus the added benefit of tax-deferral throughout the term. The money that is put into the annuity is guaranteed to earn a fixed rate of return throughout the accumulation phase of the annuity. During this phase, the money invested will continue to grow at a fixed rate (hence why it is called a *fixed* annuity).

There are basically two types of fixed annuities: **life income annuities** and **term certain fixed annuities (one to ten years).**

Life annuities pay a predetermined amount each period until the death of the policyholder. The price of a life annuity is composed of the money invested into it and the premium paid for income riders. The more insurance components on the product, or "riders," the more expensive it will be. *Straight life annuities* are the simplest form of life annuities, and their main job is to provide guaranteed-growth income to the annuitant's family after death. They are less expensive due to the fact that the only insurance component is to provide a final payout. This product, however, does not provide any form of payout throughout the life of the policy but rather after the annuitant has passed.

Fixed annuities can be categorized into **qualified** and **non-qualified annuities.** The similarity between a **qualified annuity** and a **non-qualified annuity** is they both grow tax-deferred until money is paid out or income begins. A difference between them is that the qualified annuity is fully taxable, while in the non-qualified annuity, only the growth will be taxable.

In the case of either a qualified or non-qualified fixed annuity, when the annuitant passes, the beneficiary will be responsible for the taxes on the cost of the annuity's funds. Please understand beneficiaries do not receive tax-free money if you were to leave your policy to them. This is a good example of how important it is to seek the advice of a financial professional to prevent your loved ones from being overwhelmed with tax burdens. Your financial professional should provide you with substantial options to prevent this from happening and give you even more security for your own future as well as that of your loved ones after you have passed.

Fixed Index Annuities (FIAs)[18]

A fixed index annuity (FIA) is right for you if you want the safety of a fixed annuity as well as the potential of a greater long-term growth. Fixed index annuities are a way to stack the odds in your favor against market loss since these products are licensed, regulated, and backed by the claims paying ability of the insurance company along with NOLHGA.[19] With FIAs, your money will never deplete if the market goes sour. Your account only has the opportunity to grow with guaranteed interest rates.

Remember, the best way to make money is not to lose money.

Several years ago, I had a client who moved her money from the stock market to an FIA. She was happy and satisfied with her stock portfolio, but was persuaded by family members to take on safer options. When she came into my office for her first annual review in the spring of 2008, I explained to her how her account had earned an incredible interest rate of 17 percent, but she was by no means impressed. I was dumbfounded to see this woman so underwhelmed!

When her 2009 review came around, I was scared to give her the news. The previous year she had earned a substantial amount of interest, but that year, she had earned zero. The unexpected credit freeze and downward spiral of the market meant no earned interest. People were hit so hard that year, they were filing bankruptcy and completely liquidating what was left of their accounts. To my surprise, when this woman heard the news of her zero interest, she was the happiest I had ever seen her. See, while all her friends were losing money on their accounts, she was safe. Sometimes a zero percent return like hers can be great news.

"Zero can be your hero."

Most people in the investment world are busy chasing the next "big thing," hoping to make a large return off of it. If you were to invest your money into a stock that earned more than 40 percent interest you'd be pretty excited, wouldn't you? I, for one, would be jumping for joy. But, what if the following year your investment plummeted? Yes, you can have incredible gains within a certain time frame, but you can also have incredible losses that could easily wipe out the positive returns. That means the 40 percent interest rate you once gained could turn to nothing. So, it's really not so much about what you make in a given year as much as it is about making sure you never lose any money.

A fixed index annuity is your "nest egg insurance." So, why do so many individuals leave their entire life savings completely exposed to the risk of loss without any thought to protection? I believe they simply do not know that protection *plus* the opportunity for gain exists. It does with a fixed index annuity! You reap the benefits of a market gain during its positive years, but never get hit during its negative years.

How can this be? How can any company afford to let your money increase when the market goes up but not decrease when the market goes down?

The answer is a combination of a predictable bond portfolio and what are called "options."[20] Simply put, options are tools that allow you to profit from the direction of the market. When you purchase an FIA, the majority of the premium goes toward purchasing a predictable bond portfolio that produces the same rate of interest, regardless of what the market does. The rest of the premium goes to purchase the so-called options.

Bonds provide downside protection and options provide upside growth. Your principal is guaranteed since it does not fluctuate due to market performance.

Another great benefit of an FIA is that they are tax-deferred. All annuity values accumulate on a tax-deferred basis until the money is withdrawn. This way, your money grows faster because you earn interest on money you would usually use to pay your taxes. Interest credited within an annuity is not reported to the IRS and therefore is not touched by the government until payout. Because it does not get taxed until withdrawal, receiving the funds does not subject a retiree's Social Security benefits to the destructive penalty of double taxation.

FIAs are an excellent way to guarantee lifetime income, which is one of their most powerful and beneficial aspects. An annuity is intended to grow and provide money that you can utilize in whatever form or fashion you desire in the future.

The Power of Locking in Your Interest Gains

A Fixed Index Annuity reset strategy may help you weather market downturns.

Hypothetical example of a $100,000 investment over the past ten-year period, ending 12/31/2017. Past performance is not a guarantee of future results.

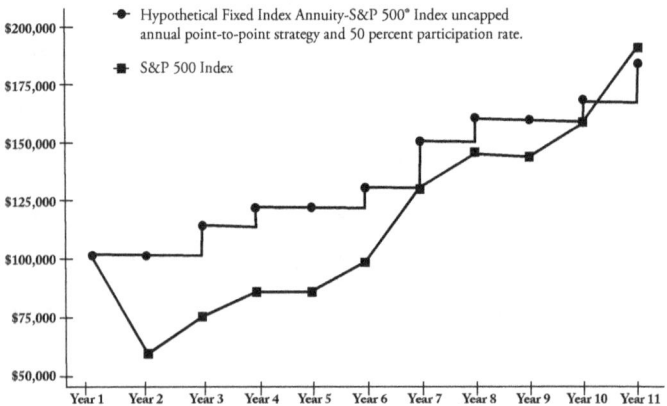

Annual reset is just one aspect of Fixed Index Annuities (FIAs), and should be part of a complete discussion including features, costs, terms, and conditions. Please talk with your financial professional for a more detailed FIA discussion.

Fixed index annuities give you the ability to turn the entire amount of the annuity into a lifetime stream of income. Insurance companies that sell FIAs offer several different annuity payment plans. For example, if you were to have a two-year FIA at 2 percent and put $100,000 into the account, at the end of the second year you would be able to pull out your principle, plus the 2 percent interest that was earned. Some accounts even allow you to pull out the interest at the end of one year. Generally, once you have an FIA in force for at least twelve months, you are allowed to take money out penalty-free. You can choose when the time is right and select the guaranteed income option that meets your needs. This can be set up so the money is either dispersed evenly throughout your life, or given to you in full at a set time.

With FIAs, you also have death benefit protection. The accumulation value of your account can go to beneficiaries if you were to pass away prior to receiving payments. Your beneficiaries then will not have to struggle through the long and expensive task of probate. They will receive the money within days or weeks, instead of months or years.

Another great benefit of most FIAs is lock-in credited interest. That means any interest gained is protected. Once the money has been credited to your annuity, it is sustained, just like the original premium.

Remember the story I told you about my client who gained a 17 percent interest in 2007 and lost nothing in the 2008 market fall? Even after the market collapsed, she still had the interest gained from the previous year. Once the money is yours, it continues to be yours.

Many fixed index annuities also pay the client a bonus on the initial purchase amount. A client who buys a $100,000 annuity with a 10 percent bonus will have an immediate account balance of $110,000. And so now, your premium amount is $110,000. Any money gained via the bonus or yearly interest is never lost.

Are there other annuity options? Yes.

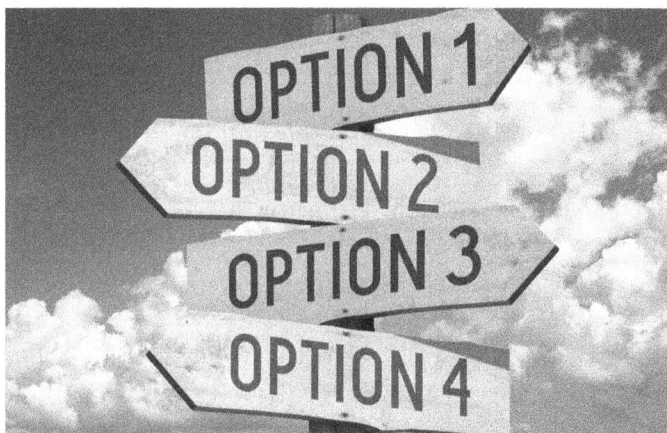

Variable Annuities[21]

A variable annuity may be right for you if you want the possibility of even greater returns and you are willing to assume more risk than with fixed or fixed index annuities. Variable annuities have the potential to grow at a higher rate than an FIA; however, there is always risk involved when investing money in the stock market.[22] Variable annuities grow based on your chosen investments and the value of these investments will vary depending on your options. You will experience both the ups and the downs of Wall Street, and you could lose money, so most people purchase optional riders to help reduce this risk. There are also fees associated with variable annuities that vary depending on your investment options.

Since variable annuities, like any annuity, come with positives and negatives, they are highly suitable for some, but certainly not for everyone. This type of annuity gives you the opportunity to make higher gains, but also increases your chances of higher losses. You are definitely taking a gamble with this product, and I do not recommend it to those looking for clear-cut safety. Variable annuities are not the safest option when looking where to put your retirement money, but for the gambler, they can mean a great deal of interest.

Like FIAs, variable annuities also let you receive payments in different ways, offer death benefits, and can be tax-deferred. The only difference between these fixed index and variable annuities is how the money is being invested.

A variable annuity has two distinct phases: an accumulation phase and a payout phase. During the accumulation phase, you make payments you can allocate to a number of different investment options. Also during this accumulation phase, you can generally transfer your money from one investment option to another without paying tax on your investment income and gains. If you were to withdraw money from your account before the age of fifty-nine and a half, you may have to pay a surrender charge and a 10 percent federal tax penalty.

Compared with mutual funds, variable annuity investment accounts often carry higher fees and expenses. Even though the accounts hold tax-deferred growth, it will eventually be taxed—it may even be taxed at the expense of your beneficiary. Guaranteed death benefits reduce your investment return. Surrender charges may be significant in early years and may continue for many years. Due to possible surrender charges and IRS tax penalties for early withdrawals, this annuity is not considered a liquid asset.

Benefits of variable annuities include: a stream of income you cannot outlive, transferring of the policy without incurring income tax liability, withdrawals for long-term health care needs, tax-deferred growth, and tax-free transfers.

Overall, the objective of an annuity is to accumulate retirement assets on a tax-deferred basis and to convert assets into an income you can never outlive.

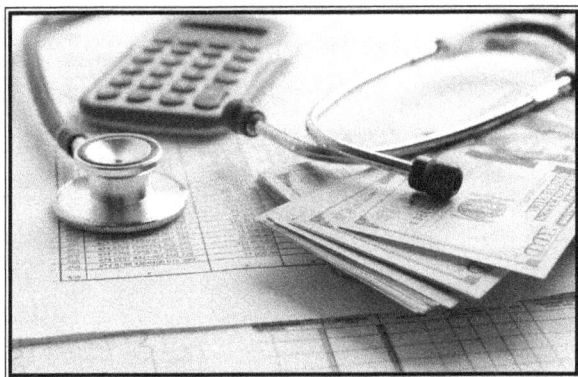

CHAPTER 6

HEALTH CARE COSTS IN RETIREMENT

One of the largest expenses for retirees is health care. It is considered the *unknown* retirement cost. Although you may live a long life, health care expenses will increase as your overall health decreases.

"Seniors spend nearly as much money on health care services and prescription drugs as they do on food."

According to a study by Fidelity Investments, an average couple of sixty-five-year-olds retiring in 2018 needed roughly $280,000 (after tax) to pay for medical expenses through retirement.[23] The health insurance scenario for retirees is scary. Medicare is running out of money and benefits are being cut. Plus, seniors have been asked to pay even more for their Medicare benefits than ever before.

According to several studies, only a fraction of the total beneficiary population has "adequate" knowledge to make an informed choice between HMOs (Health Maintenance Organization) and regular Medicare. The good news is you can have peace of mind by better understanding your health coverage options.

Medicare

Like Social Security, no retiree should rely on Medicare alone. While Medicare is very good coverage, like most health insurance plans, Medicare does not cover 100 percent of your health care costs. You will have deductibles and coinsurance and will want to evaluate the supplemental coverage options available.

Your two core options are **Original Medicare** and **Medicare Advantage** and these choices will vary based on where you live and respective plan availability.

Original Medicare

With Original Medicare, you have an option to purchase a Medicare Supplement (Medigap) policy to help cover all or some of the potential out-of-pocket costs. There are several plan options available and costs will vary based on insurance company, coverage levels, age, gender, and where you live. With Original Medicare, you will also want to consider Medicare Part D coverage to cover prescription costs. There are numerous Part D plan options available on a state-by-state basis. Medicare.gov includes a helpful "plan finder" to assist with evaluating plans. You want to be cognizant of late enrollment penalties associated with Part D plans and know these plans are only available for purchase during pre-determined eligibility periods.

Medicare Advantage

Medicare Advantage plans are simply Medicare offered by private insurance companies. Like Medicare, the plans will have co-pays, coinsurance, and deductibles that vary based on services provided. Medicare Advantage plans come in many types and associated costs can vary significantly by state and county. Most Medicare Advantage plans will include Part D prescription coverage.

To over simplify, Medicare Supplement with Part D coverage can provide the most comprehensive coverage and typically has a higher monthly cost. I often explain this as the "Pay Up Front" option. Medicare Advantage typically has lower monthly costs and will include copays and coinsurance based on services provided at hospital and physician facilities. I refer to Medicare Advantage as the "pay as you use it" option.

Keep in mind that both options require you be enrolled in Medicare Part A and Part B and you cannot have both coverages enforced at same time.

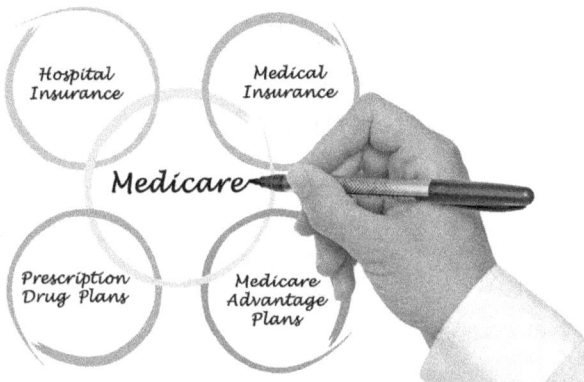

Long-term Care Insurance

When looking into health care coverage, you should also consider the chance of needing long-term care insurance. Statistics show that over half of all senior citizens will require such a policy.

With a longer life comes the possibility of needing assisted living or even skilled nursing care. The cost of assisted living averages roughly $45,536 a year, and facilities that provide skilled nursing can average more than $87,252 yearly.[24] Individuals who delay purchasing long-term coverage are generally considered high-risk and can expect to be denied coverage or be charged very high premiums. The sooner you start researching, thinking, and structuring your long-term care plans, the more options you'll have.

When considering long-term care insurance, your needs can be categorized into three groups. These resource groups—low, medium, and high—are organized according to a person's income and asset resources. When reviewing this information, again, keep in mind that costs for a skilled nursing facility and Medicaid qualification rules can vary widely from location to location. And since everyone's situation is different, the need for long-term care insurance also varies among people within the same resource group.

Low Resources Group: If you fit within this group, you have countable assets that are at or below the spend-down limits imposed by your state Medicaid rules.[25] Additionally, your typical monthly income is below the average cost of a skilled nursing (or senior care facility) in your state. Many of you within this group qualify for Medicaid without having to spend down your assets.

Medium Resources Group: If you fit within this group, you most likely will need the insurance. Your countable assets exceed the Medicaid limits, but you do not make enough money to cover the monthly costs of a care facility in your area. Compared with those in the High Resources Group, you would lack a separate source of assets to cover an extended stay in a care facility. For those of you in this group, having to come up with $7,271 per month over a long-term period could potentially deplete your estate, or create an economic hardship.

If you find yourself within this group, you should consider long-term care insurance to help secure your financial independence and preserve cherished assets for spouses and younger family members.

High Resources Group: If you are in this group, you have sufficient monthly income to cover the monthly cost of a senior care facility in your area. Or, you may have enough countable assets set aside to stay at a care facility for three to five years. However, you could still buy long-term care insurance to protect your estate from dwindling should you need it. Most importantly, long-term care insurance assures you a separate income to fund those long-term care needs.

Life Insurance

Life insurance can also help cover medical bills if you were to pass. The most important function of life insurance is to replace the earnings of a deceased loved one. Life insurance helps your family pay its regular bills and that "all-important" mortgage. And the money paid out from the life insurance policies protects your family from being bombarded with accumulated medical bills and other outstanding debts they are unable to pay.

The four major types of life insurance to consider are: **term, whole, universal,** and **variable.**

Term insurance is the simplest form of life insurance. With this policy, you purchase coverage for a specified amount of time. If you pass away during that time, your beneficiary will receive the value of the policy and they will be able to pay any pending bills you left behind.

Whole life insurance policies are a type of permanent insurance. With this policy, you purchase a fixed amount of money to cover your bills after you pass. Part of the premium builds for you a cash value that is tax-deferred each year. You can borrow against this cash accumulation fund without being taxed. The amount you pay usually does not change throughout the life of the policy.

Universal life insurance is a type of permanent insurance policy that combines term insurance with a money-market type of investment that pays a market rate of return. To get a higher return, these policies generally do not guarantee a certain rate.

Variable life insurance and **variable universal life insurance** are permanent policies that tie an investment fund to a stock or bond mutual fund investment and, therefore, returns are not guaranteed.

When considering your options for medical care expenses, remember inflation could play a huge role in the amount of money you will actually need. You need to account for the fact that things cost more over time. Necessities for living increase in price, and inflation causes your long-term savings accounts—and investments needed to cover medical care expenses—to decrease in value.

Never hesitate to ask your financial professional how inflation could affect your future. Risk that is not addressed can and will chip away at your retirement savings.

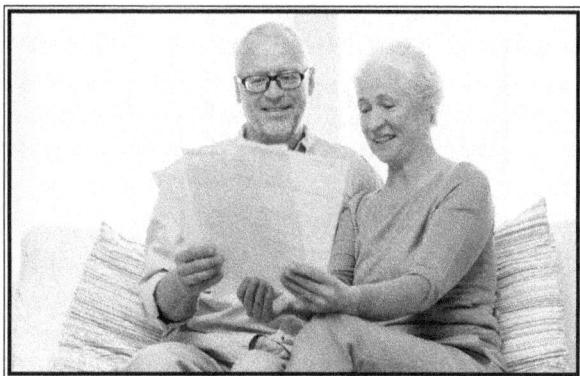

CHAPTER 7

MAKE TAXES WORK
IN YOUR FAVOR

A little planning can go a long way when it comes to taxes and your retirement. Your income is not about how much money you make, but about how much you keep after taxes. Fortunately, you can choose the right strategies to keep your taxes as low as possible if you understand how your retirement income will be taxed. Since the average retiree receives income from a wide range of sources—Social Security benefits, pensions, 401(k) plans, IRAs, annuities—knowing what is taxed and how it is taxed can make a huge difference in your retirement nest egg.

"Your income is not about how much money you make, but about how much you keep after taxes."

For example, plans you can assume are taxable include distributions from your employer's 401(k) plan, IRAs, and distributions from Roth 401(k) accounts. However, let's look at some retirement income sources below and see exactly how they will be taxed. Remember: tax planning is absolutely essential to your retirement.

Social Security
Social Security payouts may be completely or partially tax-free depending

upon your income. To plan ahead, you should know if your retirement income will cause some of your Social Security benefits to be taxed.

You can determine how portions of your Social Security benefits will be taxed using a worksheet included in the 1040 instructional booklet issued by the IRS, on page thirty-two of the 2018 edition.[26] This worksheet compares your provisional income with your benefits in the following manner:

- If your provisional income is *below* the base amounts for your filing status, then your Social Security benefits are completely non-taxable.

- If your provisional income is *between* the base amount and the additional amount, then half of your Social Security benefits over the base amount are taxable.

- If your provisional income is *over* the additional amount, 85 percent of your Social Security benefits over the additional amount are taxable.

- Overall, the taxable portion of your Social Security benefits cannot exceed 85 percent of your total benefits.

Pensions

Here's how you can determine how much of your pension payments may be taxable:

- If the distribution is from a qualified retirement plan, your pension qualifies for tax deferral. (The plan administrator or your employer can help you determine this.)
- If it is a disability pension, your pension is likely to be taxable, but if you paid the premium, the pension is *not* taxable.
- If you contributed your money from already taxed dollars, then your payouts most likely will not be taxed.

- If you pull money from your pension before the age of fifty-nine and a half, you will be taxed and may pay up to a 10 percent penalty.

All topics that follow are based on strategies to protect your retirement money from taxation.

Life Insurance Loans

Did you know that a loan based on a life insurance policy is not taxed? Let's say you borrow money to buy a new boat. The loan to buy the boat is not taxed. The boat itself may be taxed, but the loan is not. *Loans* are not taxed, *items* are. Life insurance policies can work the same way. Life insurance companies allow the policy owner to access tax-free money by using the cash value of the owner's policy as collateral for a loan. The owner avoids any tax on the money from the loan, because it is just a loan from a financial institution and not a withdrawal.

A policy owner can always take a tax-free withdrawal up to the total premiums paid into the policy, subject to surrender charges. It's tax-free because the first money allowed to come out of a life insurance policy is simply a return of the owner's total premium payments, which were previously taxed. However, if an individual wants to withdraw money above the total amount of premiums paid, then a withdrawal of this gain is taxed. The withdrawal money is taxed as income since the policy owner now withdraws money not yet taxed.

"To simplify, your money will never receive double taxation."

Whew, that was a mouthful! Some of you read that last paragraph and have absolutely no idea what I just explained to you. I know it is a lot of information. To simplify, your money will never receive double taxation. The money that started the policy was taxed, so why would the government tax you again to pull that same money out? That would be like getting a pack of gum, paying sales tax, and then receiving a 1099 form in the mail for it! The only money you will be taxed on is the interest earned, not the money that originally created the premium.

Policy Loan Provision

Policy loan provision is another option for owners of life insurance policies. Life insurance companies allow clients to take out loans *against* the cash value and not *from* the cash value. The cash value within a client's policy simply acts as collateral for this type of loan.

You may be asking, why would I want to take out this kind of a loan in my later years? Don't I get charged interest just like any other loan?

Let's say that if the interest on the loan is 4 percent and you earn 4 percent on the cash value, then the net interest rate charged is essentially zero. For those utilizing the fixed loan option, this **wash loan provision** gives continued access to their cash value, tax-free and interest-free.

The good news doesn't stop here. Since the money is distributed as a loan, it does not show up on your annual tax return. As far as the IRS is concerned, it's invisible money.

The unique tax treatment of the death benefit makes this whole loan strategy possible. Proceeds from a death benefit are income-tax-free (not estate-tax-free) without having to create a special trust. When a policy owner dies, the income-tax-free death benefit pays off the tax-free and interest-free loan. Once the loan is paid off, the leftover money is given to the beneficiary, tax-free.

Leaving an Inheritance

Now let me discuss a big mistake I see most retirees make when leaving money to their heirs.

Let's say a husband has a will, and he leaves everything to his wife or vice versa. As of 2019, every individual is allowed to pass $11.4 million of assets to his or her beneficiary without gift or estate tax.[27] However, leaving your assets to your spouse no longer excludes you from taxes. When an attorney draws up a living trust or will for you, he or she isolates the exclusion amount of assets to your heirs. This way, you can get the full benefit of your exclusion. If you are married, you get the exclusion of $11.4 million and your spouse gets his or her $11.4 million exclusion as well, making it possible that a married couple can pass a $22.8 million estate to their heirs with no estate taxes.

For those with larger estates, you should consider the idea of using some type of insurance to pay your estate taxes. For example, let's say you and your spouse have an estate of $25 million. If you are sixty-five years old or older, most likely you or your spouse will live to be eighty-five. However, if you were to die earlier, the first $22.8 million is not going to be subject to estate tax, but the other $2.2 million *will* be taxed. Let's not forget to mention that estate taxes are extremely high. On that $2.2 million, you would end up owing $880,000 in estate taxes and your heirs are the ones who have to pay it.

So, you can see why it is important to look into insurance policies that can protect you from this misfortune. And, keep in mind that in order for the policy to be protected from taxes, it has to stay in force until the insured's death. If the policy cancels for any reason, then all of the gain from a tax-free loan will suddenly become taxable. To ensure that your life insurance policy stays in force, make sure not to take out too much money, run the income stream well past the average life expectancy, and review your policy annually.

Annuities

As I mentioned before, annuities can be a great way to protect yourself from taxes. Annuity income is considered a combination of return of principal plus earnings, and only the earnings are taxed as ordinary income for non-qualified accounts. Qualified accounts, except Roth IRAs, are taxed fully. When working to build your retirement assets, the tax-deferred growth from annuities can help protect you against the risk of outliving your retirement savings.

Fixed annuities offer defined growth, principal, and interest—all free from taxes until withdrawal. However, if you purchase an annuity with pre-tax dollars from a product such as a 401(k) or an IRA, the entire payout may be subject to income taxes. This is because the money contributed initially was never taxed.

"Annuities can also help reduce or eliminate the tax on your Social Security benefits."

As we explained earlier, taxpayers today can pay up to 85 percent of their Social Security income. The IRS calculates the tax on your Social Security income based on your total income from all sources. However, any income you earn on an annuity that is left to accumulate does not appear on your current tax returns. If you shelter enough income in annuities and bring your income below the threshold, you then pay no tax on your Social Security income.

Equity-indexed annuities can offer tax deferral as well as some market-risk protection, a minimum interest rate guarantee, probate savings, and guaranteed minimum income payment for life. The interest earnings for these annuities are based upon the growth in an accepted equity index, such as the S&P 500 Index, Dow Jones Industrial Average, and Russell 2000. The interest rate applied to these annuities is based upon the overall movement of the index. Many annuities will also base the interest rate upon a pre-determined percentage of the market movement.

Tax-free Bonds

Many people turn to tax-free bonds when looking for other ways to produce tax-free income. Tax-free bonds are popular, but actually you can get a higher cash flow from insurance companies.

One excellent source of tax-free income is an **immediate annuity.** In exchange for the premium payment, the insurance company pays the annuity owner a cash payment for life or for a certain number of years. Each payment is comprised of interest and principal as determined by an actuarial calculation, or a calculation that deals specifically with financial risk and uncertainty. The principal portion of the payment is not subject to income taxation. Once the owner has recovered his or her investment, the remaining payments will be taxed as ordinary income.

Let me give you an example: Mr. Jones is seventy years old and has a portfolio of $500,000 in municipal bonds earning 4.35 percent, tax-free. He receives $21,750 of annual tax-free income. He then decides to cash in his tax-free bonds and pay a premium of $500,000 to an insurance company in order to buy an immediate fixed annuity. His yearly cash payment from the annuity is $42,540 per year. Seventy-three percent of this is taxed as the tax-free portion of the annuity. For tax purposes, the IRS considers return of your principal, your life expectancy, and the expected return. After taxes, Mr. Jones will now have $39,668 to spend. His spendable cash increased annually by $17,918 when he chose the immediate fixed annuity over the tax-free bonds.

Even though Mr. Jones's cash flow did increase by using the immediate annuity, this annuity is not for everyone. An immediate annuity will not leave anything for your heirs unless you purchase from a company that offers a refund feature. This refund feature typically reduces the size of the monthly annuity payment and sometimes the amount of the refund may be reduced by surrender charges. Therefore, the immediate annuity is generally better suited for people who want to increase their lifetime cash flow and are not concerned with leaving money to their heirs.

Distributions

Taking smaller distributions is another great way to preserve your retirement funds and decrease your taxations. All too often I see clients taking out more money than they should. It is great to have new goals and dreams in retirement, but if those dreams require more money than you originally planned to spend, you may need to rethink what you're doing.

Everything must be strategic when it comes to your retirement money. For example, it would probably not be wise to use your saved money to buy a yacht. Though we all want to sit on the edge of a boat sipping margaritas, if a yacht-life was not in your original budget, maybe don't be so unrealistic. Even worse, if you were to take out more money from a retirement policy than you were allotted, you could be looking at a great deal of taxation—and even penalties!

Let's say you have two pots of money: regular money and retirement money. When you spend $1 of regular money, the cost to you is $1. When you spend

$1 of your retirement money, the cost to you is more like $1.54 because of the federal income tax you may have to pay on the amount you withdraw. Therefore, if you want to reduce your taxes, consider not taking out more than the required distribution from your retirement money.

Many people think they should never spend their principal, but from an income-tax standpoint, you would possibly be better off financially if you did. It could be better to spend part of your regular assets first, and take advantage of the tax-deferral benefits associated with IRAs and qualified retirement plans. Your lifetime tax bill could be less, or at least you would defer taxes for many years.

Roth IRAs

Roth IRA contributions are not taxed at the time you make them, because your contributions come from post-tax income. Roth IRAs do not receive the tax break that pre-tax retirement accounts such as traditional IRAs and 401(k) plans receive. Pre-tax retirement accounts are funded with income that has not been taxed. These plans avoid paying tax today, but must pay income tax when the funds are withdrawn in retirement.

Despite the lack of its tax break today, a Roth IRA may end up being a great investment vehicle to minimize your taxes over a long period of time. The further out your retirement date, the greater chance your personal income-tax rates will increase. If you lock in paying a certain rate today and your personal tax rate is higher at retirement, then using a Roth IRA will have saved you money. Investment income earned inside a Roth IRA is not reported on your annual tax return, and does not require minimum distributions. Roth IRAs can also be handed down to heirs, tax-free.

With or without a tax break, another benefit of using a Roth IRA (over pre-tax investment accounts like traditional IRAs) is you can withdraw your contributions (not earnings) at any point without paying taxes or fees. But keep in mind, there are income restrictions for being eligible to fund a Roth IRA, and losses in a Roth IRA are tax-deductible only if cashed out completely. In 2019, maximum contributions per year are $6,000 if you are under age fifty, and $7,000 if you are age fifty or older.[28]

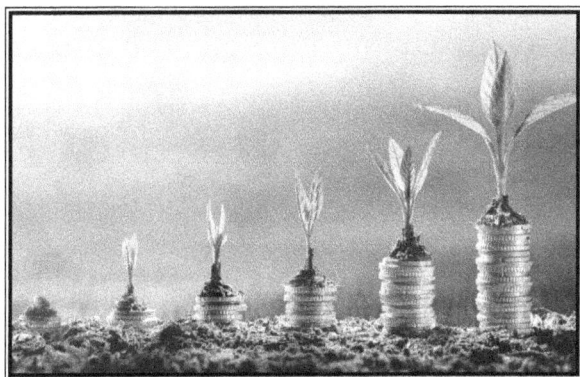

INCOME TO LAST

One question no one can answer is "how long will you live?" We all want our income to last—especially since the fastest-growing group of people who file for bankruptcy is senior citizens.[29]

Nearly three in five retirees will run out of money if they maintain their pre-retirement lifestyle without reducing their spending by nearly 25 percent. Cutting down on what you spend will obviously help to stretch your income, but you must also proactively manage your investment options and savings to effectively make your income last.

The 4 Percent Rule

For more than a generation, the "4 percent rule" seemed safe and appropriate. The rule stated if you did not withdraw more than 4 percent of your retirement nest egg each year, you would have enough money to last at least thirty years into retirement.

"The 4 percent rule seemed appropriate in the past, but may not be considered so safe today."

The rule was created in 1993 by Bill Bengen. Mr. Bengen tested many different withdrawal percentages to see which one would allow savings to last at least thirty years. (Many do not know Bill

Bengen actually found that 4.5 percent was ideal, but the rule kept its 4 percent name regardless.) Though Bill Bengen may have been on to something years ago, the 4 percent rule simply does not hold true for today's retiree who wants to avoid outliving his or her money. In the low-yield world we all face in today's economy, many financial professionals reject the rule and turn to other means of saving.

Mr. Bengen's 4 percent rule does not acknowledge new economic realities with its potentially prolonged low returns. Michael Finke, a professor in the department of personal financial planning at Texas Tech University said, "We've never had an extended period where rates of returns on bonds have been so low and valuation on stocks so high."[30]

The 60/40 portfolio allocation is based on the 4 percent rule, and many advisors recommend moving away from that type of allocation.[31] Interest rates today are nothing like what they used to be, and with most investments, you certainly can't depend on them.

So, if you want a more certain future, I would recommend putting money into an annuity product. Since annuities pay a yearly income that kicks in later in life, they ensure you will not run out of income in your later years. If you take up to half of your retirement savings from 401(k)s and IRAs and put that amount into annuity accounts, those funds will provide you with guaranteed income after retirement.

Portfolio vs. Annuity

Examples using two hypothetical people illustrate for us two different strategies for making income last through retirement. Let's say Sarah withdraws money solely from an investment portfolio, whereas John withdraws money from both an investment portfolio and an annuity account.

Sarah relies on just regular withdrawals from her portfolio to fill her income gap. She risks depleting her portfolio early due to inflation and down-market conditions. Her money is not protected. In the hands of a roller coaster economy, more than likely Sarah's portfolio will not generate enough money to last. Her money could potentially not gain enough interest to beat inflation, and it wouldn't protect her if something were to happen to the market. (No one can predict market performance.)

Now let's imagine that by some miracle, Sarah is able to pull through in saving for her retirement by decreasing her overall debt expense, and the market has an excellent few years. Luck is on her side! The markets are booming for her and she never loses a penny. Sarah then decides because her luck is so high, she can start pulling out money from her investments early. She is no longer budgeting for the future, but Sarah is sure the market will support her either way. Unfortunately, Sarah didn't take into account that the market could drop or that the money she was using was necessary for her future.

> *"Living off of luck is one of the most dangerous things you can do in retirement and can almost guarantee you won't have income to last."*

Now, John, on the other hand, takes money from his portfolio as well as from his annuity account, which is guaranteed to grow interest and never deplete. His fixed annuity pays a set amount each year. John wisely does not want to lose money or security and is willing to give up access to some of his savings.

Money from annuities is money John can depend on. Even though he has money invested in the market, he can rely on the annuity completely if something happens to the market. The combination of an investment portfolio plus an annuity gives John guaranteed income to help cover essential expenses.

John also has IRAs (including a Roth IRA) plus a 401(k). Because John is smart, he pulls funds first from taxable accounts since they may be taxed at a lower long-term capital gains rate. This gives John's tax-advantaged accounts more time to build up without taxes dragging them down. The result? He ends up with more money for retirement. If he waits until the age of seventy and a half, John can then withdraw funds from those tax-advantaged accounts and avoid taxation.

Sadly, Sarah is "livin' on a prayer" as Bon Jovi would say. Depending solely on an undependable market, she hoped for the best and accumulated the worst. Sarah never stopped to re-adjust her retirement planning.

Conversely, John did plan properly for a while, but now he's decided he's done with all that. John is tired of thinking about finances. He loses control of his accounts because he is no longer proactive. John does not know whether he needs to scale back or withdraw more money. Even worse, the market status could leave John in a heap of a mess. John needs to schedule a yearly review with his financial professional in order to not overlook crucial decisions.

Both John and Sarah should make sure they are not living above their means. Hitting retirement doesn't mean they can start splurging. It has always been a running joke to "spend your child's inheritance," but by doing so, John and Sarah—and all of us—could also be tapping into crucial retirement funds. Maybe John decides to buy a fancy new car on a whim, and Sarah up and decides to take a cruise to the Greek islands. They are not taking into account any unexpected expenses down the road.

And, excessive spending habits certainly won't leave money for their heirs.

If anything, Sarah and John both need to reduce expenses—not create more. If they do that, they will extend the lives of their incomes and their own financial peace of mind.

Reducing Expenditures

Housing is generally the biggest expense for a family. This cost alone makes up one-third of the average American household budget.[32] The easiest way to reduce housing expenses is to downsize. Smaller houses for both Sarah and John would not only reduce mortgage payments, but also help save money on utilities, maintenance, and a never-ending amount of property bills. They could also benefit from moving closer to family for support. In today's environment, taking on a modest mortgage and then paying it off should be the goal. If John and Sarah were to downsize their homes, they could use the equity to help fund retirement income via a reverse mortgage.

Getting out of debt, or at least downsizing debt, is another way to provide financial security down the road. It is imperative to reduce debt before retirement. Debt does two things to your income: it increases risk and robs you of cash flow. If Sarah or John were facing overwhelming credit card bills, they should focus on paying their debts with the highest interest rates first. They could also consider consolidating their debt on a card that offers a zero percent interest rate.

Budgeting

Setting up a budget is also pertinent to making Sarah's and John's incomes last.

Their first step in budgeting is to make a detailed monthly expense report based on their current standard of living. Next, they can create another budget based on the retirement lifestyle they decide they want and include a plan to keep expenses low. Just because they are retiring doesn't mean they should start spending their money on unnecessary items. Sarah and John should save that kind of spending for the money they win from the lottery!

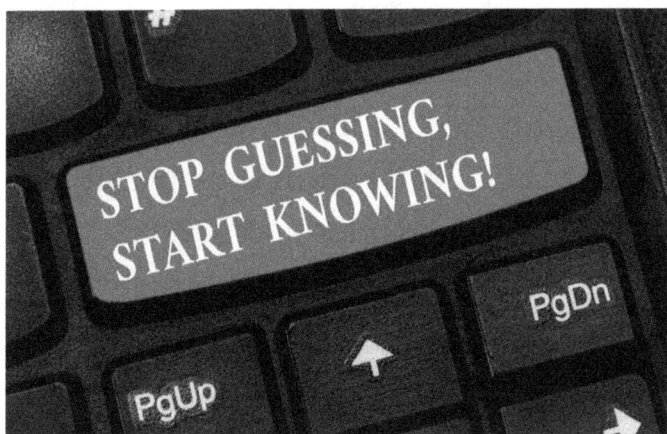

In conclusion, putting money into investment portfolios as well as annuity products can ensure income that will last. It is important to make sure the market is working for you, not the other way around. Taking enough risk with a valid amount of security will give you a return you'll be able to live off of for a long time. Be cautious, however, of losing track of how you've invested, or forgetting to review accounts with your financial professional annually. This error alone could leave you wishing you had.

When it comes to income, do you want to guess or to know? Most importantly, think of the following question, "is the reward worth the risk?" This article I wrote for *forbes.com* in 2018 will give you perspective on this very important question.

Featured on *forbes.com*
Article by: Dolph Janis
Published: March 2018

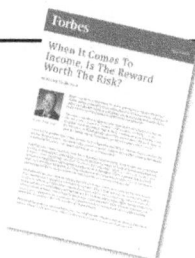

When It Comes To Income, Is The Reward Worth The Risk?

Imagine you are at the roulette table in a casino and are given an opportunity for your lifetime savings of $500,000. You have two choices, A and B. If you choose option A, you will receive a monthly paycheck of $2,000 for the rest of your life. With option B, you could receive a monthly paycheck of $5,000 for the rest of your life.

The choice seems obvious, right? Not quite. If you read it correctly, option B does not offer the certainty of option A. The word 'could' expresses possibility—and only possibility. That means there is a risk involved—a spin on the wheel. If it lands on red, you will receive the $5,000 monthly paycheck for the rest of your life, but if it lands on black, you receive nothing. Now, what do you do? Is the reward worth the risk?

That is the BIG question! Since I began focusing on income planning in 2005, four out of five clients I meet face this decision: the known versus the unknown, the certainty of a paycheck versus the possibility of making more money in the market. We refer to it as 'income planning' vs. 'income guessing.'

One of the most common fears individuals have is that of outliving their money. Think of it this way: in retirement, you 'pay' yourself instead of someone paying you. So, you have to consider the many unknowns attached not only to retirement, but also through retirement. For example, how long will you live? You could live ten, twenty, thirty, or more years in retirement! That is why longevity is considered one of the biggest risks in retirement. How much will your health care cost? What will inflation do? These are just a few of the unknowns. So, again I ask, when it comes to your savings and the income you need for the rest of your life, is the reward worth the risk?

Continued on next page

In my years of experience, I have seen many individuals worry more about how much money they have to retire, rather than how much income they will receive in retirement. Many of them have not even considered longevity, health care, inflation, and all the other unknowns associated with the cost of living during retirement. When you focus on income, you can eliminate many fears and worries. Social Security, pensions, and income annuities are the primary sources of lifetime income (based on the strength of the government, the company you worked for, and the insurance company). So, if you could plan for a monthly income for as long as you live, no matter how long, would that take away your fear? This is what I call 'income planning.'

Even though the phrase 'income planning' is quite clear, a high number of individuals go for option B. They choose the risk, hoping to make more money without looking at the consequences; they are 'income guessing.'

As I often say on my radio show, "The best way to make money is not to lose money." That is why working with an income strategist makes a lot of sense.

When it comes to income planning, there are many strategies out there. Finding the best strategies for you is the job of the income planner you work with. Keep in mind that it is more important to focus on how much income you will have coming in, rather than how much money you have going into retirement. You can count on lifetime income; it will always be there. With assets, you are dealing with the unknown.

In building your portfolio, besides the main question, "Do I want to live with no worries or fears about my finances?" you also have to ask yourself the following: "Would I like to leave my loved ones a legacy?" and "Is keeping control of my funds important to me?" These are questions that shape your financial future. Your path will be unique. What is right for one person is not necessarily right for another person. Finding what is best for you and your family for your financial future should be one of your priorities. Your portfolio has to be what is comfortable for you, be it protecting it all or deciding to risk some in hopes of making more. To make decisions, you must ponder the consequences and ask yourself, "Is the reward of making more money worth the risk of losing money?"

Now, imagine this scenario: You admit your fear of running out of money in retirement and take the first step to see a financial professional. After a couple of meetings, they offer you a solution to your concern. The solution is everything you were looking for. Now, you have to commit to that solution. Sadly, this is where many people fail; they procrastinate making the decision. Procrastinating can change your financial outcome!

If you, along with your financial professional, have done the work, cleverly decided to income plan, designed the best portfolio for you, and found a solution to your financial worries about retirement, is it worth the wait? No, it is not worth that wait! Do not procrastinate. Think of the reward: added peace of mind.

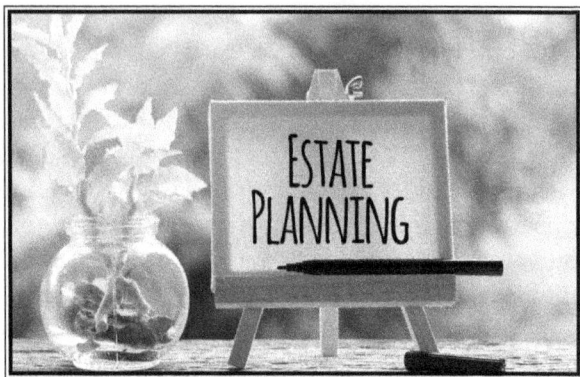

CHAPTER 9
ESTATE PLANNING

Everyone has an estate no matter how large or how modest it may be. No matter your net worth, it is important to have an estate plan. Too many individuals put off estate planning because they think they don't own enough, feel they have plenty of time, or don't know where to begin. Good estate planning means the most to families with modest assets because they can afford to lose the least.

Your assets include everything you own—whether it is your investments, retirement savings, insurance policies, and real estate or business interests. Estate planning entails determining where all of your assets will be dispersed after you have passed, but it is much more than that.

Estate planning can and should include:

- an inventory of assets,
- a will left to heirs,
- possible trusts,
- instructions regarding your own care if you were to become disabled,
- listed guardians for minors,
- means to provide for loved ones after you have passed,
- ways to minimize taxes and legal fees that could be left to family members.

If you do not have a predetermined estate plan set in place, the state will automatically set one for you—a plan you may not necessarily agree with. The court will decide how your assets are dispersed, where minors go, what happens to investments, and insurance policies. Unless you want absolutely no say in what happens after you have passed, estate planning is essential.

Estate planning begins with a will or trust. The disadvantage to a will is that it means probate.[33] Any assets titled in your name or directed by your will must go through your state's probate process before they can be distributed to your heirs. This process can take years and cost a great deal of money, and even joint ownership cannot guarantee your escape from probate.

Most people prefer a revocable living trust. With such a trust you avoid probate, court costs, and provide maximum privacy of your assets. A living trust is more expensive than a will, but more cost efficient in the long run because you can avoid court fees.

If the tasks involved in estate planning seem too much on your own, an attorney and a tax advisor can help you. An attorney can guide you through the creation of the fundamental estate planning documents like a will, health care options, and durable power of attorney. A tax advisor can help you with any potential tax issues.

You take charge of making the decisions, but an attorney and tax advisor help you to think through the process and better understand the complexities of estate planning. They can help you write your will and/or trusts in such a way that makes your wishes clear and mistake-free. An attorney can also help you make any changes you wish to make to your plan down the road.

Estate planning is all about maximizing your assets. It's important to get legal or tax advice on how assets will pass to your beneficiaries. The best options vary based on the kind of asset and its size. Financial and tax professionals ensure you lose as little as possible to taxes, court fees, or any other additional costs.

As stated in Chapter 7, a big part of maximizing your assets is minimizing taxes. Since federal tax on estates is one of the highest forms of taxation, minimizing this taxation is essential. Estate and inheritance taxes are generally based on the value of the taxable estate and are paid before the assets are distributed to beneficiaries. One option is to use the gift tax exemption to transfer assets while you are still alive and maximize what your beneficiaries will receive.

Besides an inventory list of all of your physical assets and accounts, estate planning should include a list of debts and credit cards, including everything from existing mortgages, auto loans, open credit cards with and without balances, to any other form of debt you may have. Never leave out the little things when planning your estate. The little things could mean the difference in your heirs' potential to carry on your legacy. For example, a list of organizations you belong to might be important to your beneficiaries. Perhaps it would also be important to leave information regarding how to contact your financial professionals and attorneys.

Below are three examples of estate planning based on clients with whom I have had the pleasure of working. I hope you can learn from their mistakes as well as from the things they did right.

First, let's talk about David. David was divorced and planned to leave his assets to his son, Jason. David had mentally planned a lot of things regarding his estate, but he never had anything "written in stone." David had always said he would do it later. He had planned to seek a professional advisor regarding his estate, but he unfortunately passed away before he had the chance.

Not only did Jason expect some of the estate, but David's ex-wife did as well. No longer was David able to decide what would happen. Jason wanted his father's hunting guns in particular, but there was no proof these items were left to him. Sadly, state laws intervened and created an estate plan for David without any regards to what he would have wanted. This is exactly what happens with probate; only the court can decide what happens to those guns.

Another example is Sam. Sam had no family left and zero heirs. Despite this fact, he did have two cats and a dog. Sam spent the majority of his time with his pets. Though he loved them unconditionally, he never thought about what would happen to his pets after he passed.

Sam forgot to consider the three most important things in his life! Had Sam set up a pet trust to care for his animals, he would have been able to rest assured, knowing they would be taken care of.

Now, I know this example may seem a bit silly, but it does show how important it is to plan every aspect of your estate. Not one detail should be left out. I'm not saying you should leave everything to Mr. Whiskers, your cat, but you must consider every part of your life—even your pets.

Susan is a prime example of how to do estate planning well. After her husband passed away, Susan was diligent in updating her end-of-life documents. She updated her will and obtained a Power of Attorney to ensure all her needs were met, and she put her son in charge of managing her financial affairs.

She included in a file all the information for her lawyer, stockbroker, accountant, and insurance agent. She also put her son in charge of all her medical decisions in case she was no longer able to make those decisions for herself. Susan also left enough money to cover her funeral costs and bills. She even went so far as to discuss what she wanted to wear at her funeral.

In conclusion, be sure to ask yourself the following questions when planning your estate:

- Who do you want to inherit your assets?
- Who do you want to handle your financial affairs in case you are incapacitated?
- Who do you want to make medical decisions for you if you become unable to make them for yourself?

CONCLUSION

Now that you understand you can't just cross the bridge to retirement blindfolded, you must prepare to cross it safely and securely. Planning is the key. Moreover, if you are already in retirement, you can benefit from learning how to keep it stress-free. The realities of retirement are changing, and I hope you received a lot of necessary information by reading this book. Today is the day to start planning for your future.

Many Americans believe there is a retirement crisis happening now and fear they are either unprepared or underprepared. With proper guidance from a financial professional, and by maintaining a positive outlook, you can rest assured your retirement years will be the best of your life. Today is the day to take a more active role in planning for—and protecting—your future.

> *"I love and often use the phrase: 'A failure to plan is a plan for failure.'"*

Preparing for retirement involves budgeting, saving, and understanding your future needs. No one knows what their future will hold, so it is important to plan accordingly. You may end up living to 110!

The 4 Cs are a great place to start asking yourself the necessary questions. After reviewing the 4 Cs, you can then decide how to divide your money between today, tomorrow, and never money.

What you once thought you knew about retirement is certainly not the same. Social Security can no longer be your only asset. Like many Americans, you are facing one of the biggest retirement income challenges in history! Reliable sources of income (like Social Security) are disappearing as life expectancies are rising. Even worse, the 4 percent rule is practically obsolete in today's economy. In light of these statistics, increased personal responsibility for retirement is pertinent.

In a world of financial insecurities, trying to save money may make you even more vulnerable to market turbulence. Depending on your risk tolerance, there are many products that can provide steady income in retirement without the worry of loss. Remember, unless you are a high risk-taker, you should never rely on the stock market to ensure financial success.

Annuity-like solutions are gaining relevance and appeal. They can be a valuable addition to your overall retirement strategy as they offer tax-deferred growth while you save for retirement, and dependable income after you retire. Many annuities also provide principal protection, and some can be customized to provide inflation protection, enhanced death benefit, and lifetime income. Other options, such as riders, can also be readily available for an additional cost. Additionally, annuities can help provide for your heirs after you have passed.

As you now know, there are many different types of annuities, and the only way to fully know which one is best suited for you is to speak with a financial professional in your area. Annuities are complex products that should be discussed in full.

Planning for tomorrow could also mean planning for rising health care costs, inflation, needs of beneficiaries, future medical expenses, after-life expenses, and so much more. It is up to you and your financial professional to thoroughly plan according to your potential needs. My hope is this book helps you to think through some of those needs, so nothing is overlooked.

Now is the time to start planning for tomorrow. I hope you found my book to be of benefit, and may your journey toward retirement be a pleasant one. Take control of your future and take the first step today, so you can easily cross the bridge to retirement tomorrow. In closing, I want to leave you with the following article I wrote for *Annuity 123* in 2016, which stresses the importance of discipline and planning in this once-in-a-lifetime process of retiring.

Featured on *Annuity 123*
Article by: Dolph Janis
Published: March 2016

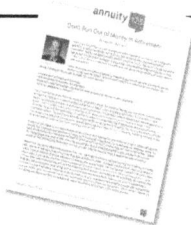

Don't Run Out of Money in Retirement

Have you ever awoken at night and started worrying about running out of money when you're in or entering retirement? Does the fear of losing what you have saved for retirement due to changing markets concern you? If so, you're not alone. A large number of baby boomers have this feeling on a daily basis. I have been working with clients for over eleven years, and these concerns are brought up in just about every meeting or conversation I have with clients.

When looking at the different places to invest money, individuals look into stocks, bonds, mutual funds, and real estate. Why wouldn't they? Those are what people always talk about. I challenge you to ask yourself, can those vehicles:

- Protect your principle and nest egg?
- Provide protection against the unknown?
- Guarantee a worst-case scenario with an optional lifetime income payment?
- Give you added peace of mind?

If you said "no" to more than one of these, you are not alone. The common feeling you have when trying to make money from your own mon-

Continued on next page

ey is similar to that of Las Vegas—and why it's so successful. It's a 'greed vs. fear' factor. Speaking from experience as a previous casino dealer in Las Vegas, where the odds are stacked against you to win, most individuals play without thinking of the potential outcome and end up losing in the process—motivated by greed! The others play so cautiously, never knowing when to get aggressive versus conservative—motivated by fear! The same goes with the stock market. To quote Kenny Rogers: "You have to know when to hold 'em, know when to fold 'em, know when to walk away, and know when to run." Timing the market is not easy; it can be costly and can prevent you from running out of money.

Discipline and planning are major factors when it comes to preparing for your retirement years. When talking with clients, the most common question is, "How much money will I have when I'm in retirement?" Whereby, unlike the past, it is actually more important for them to think about how much income they will have in retirement. People are living longer and need to start planning accordingly. Utilize what is available to you, and don't fall into the 'greed vs. fear' philosophy. Remember this key phrase: "The best way to make money is not to lose money!"

When I ask my clients what their top three fears are, the majority of them say that running out of money is number one, second is talking in front of a group of people, and third is death. It amazes me that more people are afraid to talk in front of a bunch of people and have no money than actual death. This is a common subject I talk with clients about daily. In doing this, it comes down to preparation and discipline. Layer your funds so you always have liquid money, keep your money protected, and have optional fixed annuity contracts that can provide an optional income that you can never outlive to go along with your Social Security payments (so they can be used as supplemental income, the way they were intended). And last, make sure you have money set aside for unexpected emergencies that just might arise during your retirement. No need to take risks. Protect and grow your future without the worry of running out of money! Take the guesswork out of retirement, and consult a retirement planner.

ABOUT THE AUTHOR

Randall 'Dolph' Janis is the founder and President of Clear Income Strategies Group, LLC. Mr. Janis is an advanced financial professional who has been trained in comprehensive cutting-edge retirement income techniques. Since 2005, he has helped hundreds of baby boomers fully navigate through market volatility and corrections. Most importantly, Mr. Janis has helped his clients keep on the safe path to retirement and then retire (and stay retired!) comfortably. Mr. Janis believes in planning for the known versus guessing against the unknown. He preaches, *"the best way to make money is not to lose money,"* by educating individuals and clients about the many options and strategies involved in retirement.

Mr. Janis has been on the radio since 2010 and hosts the Income Strategies Radio show in Charlotte, North Carolina. He has written articles published in *Forbes Magazine, Fortune, Money,* and *Annuity 123.* He has been featured in articles and appeared in the *Wall Street Journal, US News & World Report,* Investopedia, Nasdaq, CBS, Bankrate, MSN Money, Good Call, Wise Break, Yahoo, *The Kansas City Star,* SafeBee, Fox News, Discover, *Huffpost,* CB Insights, WBT-TV, Credit Card Guide, TheStreet, Spectrum News, and more.

Mr. Janis and his company are proud members of the National Ethics Association as well as A+ members of the BBB (Better Business Bureau) of the Carolinas.

DISCLOSURES

reviewed, approved, endorsed, or authorized by the Social Security Administration.

The material in this book is intended for informational purposes only. One might potentially use a variety of different investment and/or insurance products in planning for retirement. Everyone should consult with their own financial professional to assist them in determining which options are most suitable for them, based on their specific situation and objectives.

Any mention within the pages of this book regarding a particular product or strategy as a means of addressing retirement income concerns is not meant to be constructed as a definitive, only, or best available option for that purpose.

The S&P 500® is designed to be a leading indicator of US equities and is meant to reflect risk/return characteristics of the large cap sector. It is not available for direct investment.

For any given financial concern, there can be multiple solutions that might utilize a number of different investment or insurance products. If the author demonstrates any bias toward a given product, strategy, or security, it is because the author feels strongly about the merits of that vehicle in this application. As always, you are strongly encouraged to weigh all your options and meet with a qualified, licensed individual in your area to assist you in determining your best option(s).

Any transaction that involves a recommendation to liquidate a securities product, including those within an IRA, 401(k), or other retirement plan, for the purchase of an annuity or for other similar purposes, can be conducted only by individuals who are appropriately licensed and currently affiliated with a properly registered broker/dealer or registered investment advisor. If your financial professional does not hold the appropriate registration, please consult with your own broker/dealer representative or investment advisor representative for guidance on your securities holdings.

Please note that the use of terms similar to, or related to the word "guarantee," including all variations thereof when describing an insurance product, including fixed index annuities, are based entirely on the fact that any contractual guarantees within the insurance product are backed solely by the financial strength and claims-paying ability of the insurance company that issues the contract or policy.

The contents of this book should not be taken as financial advice, or as an offer to buy or sell any securities, fund, or financial instruments. Any illustrations or examples presented are hypothetical and do not take into account your particular investment objectives, financial situation, or needs, and are not suitable for all persons. Any investments and/or investment strategies mentioned involve risk, including the possible loss of principal. There is no assurance that any investment strategy will achieve its objectives. No portion of this content should be construed as an offer or solicitation for the purchase or sale of any security. The contents of this book should not be taken as an endorsement or recommendation of any particular company or individual, and no responsibility can be taken for inaccuracies, omissions, or errors.

The author and publisher specifically disclaim responsibility for any liability, loss, or risk, personal or otherwise, that is incurred as a consequence, directly or indirectly, of the use and application of any contents of this book.

Trademarks: All terms mentioned in this book that are known to be or are suspected of being trademarks or service marks have been appropriately capitalized. The publisher cannot attest to the accuracy of this information. Use of a term in this book should not be regarded as affecting the validity of any trademark or service mark.

The author does not assume any responsibility for actions or non-actions taken by people who have read this book, and no one shall be entitled to a claim for detrimental reliance based upon any information provided or expressed herein. Your use of any information provided does not constitute any type of contractual relationship between yourself and the provider(s) of this information. The author hereby disclaims all responsibility and liability for all use of any information provided in his book. The materials here are not to be interpreted as establishing an attorney-client or any other relationship between the reader and the author or his firm.

Although great effort has been expended to ensure only the most meaningful resources are referenced in these pages, the author does not endorse, guarantee, or warranty the accuracy, reliability, or thoroughness of any referenced information, product, or service. Any opinions, advice, statements, services, offers, or other information or content expressed or made available by third parties are those of the author(s) or publisher(s) alone.

References to other sources of information do not constitute a referral, endorsement, or recommendation of any product or service. The existence of any particular reference is simply intended to imply potential interest to the reader.

Hypothetical example(s) are for illustrative purposes only and are not intended to represent the past or future performance of any specific investment.

ENDNOTES

1 https://www.allianzlife.com/-/media/files/allianz/documents/ent_991_n.pdf?
   la=en&hash+1DB3AED9D8744BF645AAE77C04BC5A0864E52F7E
2 https://www.ssa.gov/planners/lifeexpectancy.html
3 Rebalancing/Reallocating can entail transaction costs and tax
   consequences that should be considered when determining a
   rebalancing/reallocation strategy.
4 https://www.allianzlife.com/-/media/files/allianz/documents/ent_1340_n.
   pdf?la=en&hash=EE9BB2CD6B1848F3AABFAE9495947AF7E08576D4.
   Gary Bhojwani of Allianz Life Insurance Company of North America
   originally created the 4 Cs of successful retirement income strategies. It is
   only being used in *Cross the Bridge to Retirement* for perspective purposes.
   Additionally, all graphs are from studies conducted by Allianz.
5 http://www.ncsl.org/research/health/health-insurance-premiums.aspx
6 Fixed Annuities are long-term insurance contacts and there is a surrender
   charge imposed generally during the first five to seven years that you own
   the annuity contract. Withdrawals prior to age fifty-nine and a half may
   result in a 10 percent IRS tax penalty, in addition to any ordinary income
   tax. Any guarantees of the annuity are backed by the financial strength of
   the underlying insurance company.
7 Please consider the investment objectives, risks, charges, expenses, and
   your need for death-benefit coverage carefully before investing. The
   prospectus, which contains this and other information about the variable
   life policy and the underlying investment options, can be obtained from
   your financial professional. Be sure to read the prospectus carefully before
   deciding whether to invest. The investment return and principal value
   of the variable life policy are not guaranteed. Variable life sub-accounts
   fluctuate with changes in market conditions. The principal may be
   worth more or less than the original amount invested when the policy is
   surrendered. Any guarantees offered are backed by the financial strength
   of the insurance company.
8 Indexed Universal Life Insurance is an insurance contract that, depending
   on the contract, may offer a guaranteed annual interest rate and some
   participation growth, if any, of a stock market index. Such contracts have
   substantial variation in terms, costs of guarantees, and features, and may
   cap participation or returns in significant ways. Any guarantees offered are
   backed by the financial strength of the insurance company, not an outside
   entity. Investors are cautioned to carefully review an indexed universal life
   insurance for its features, costs, risks, and how the variables are calculated.

9   The investment return and principal value of the variable annuity investment options are not guaranteed. Variable annuity sub-accounts fluctuate with changes in market conditions. The principal may be worth more or less than the original amount invested when the annuity is surrendered.

10 Indexed annuities are insurance contracts that, depending on the contract, may offer a guaranteed annual interest rate and some participation growth, if any, of a stock market index. Such contracts have substantial variation in terms, costs of guarantees, and features, and may cap participation or returns in significant ways. Any guarantees offered are backed by the financial strength of the insurance company. Surrender charges apply if not held to the end of the term. Withdrawals are taxed as ordinary income and, if taken prior to age fifty-nine and a half, a 10 percent federal tax penalty. Investors are cautioned to carefully review an indexed annuity for its features, costs, risks, and how the variables are calculated.

11 Life insurance can also benefit your loved ones in other ways as well in the form of estate tax coverage, business succession planning, income replacement, and mortgage and debt coverage.

12 Not associated with or endorsed by the Social Security Administration or any other government agency.

13 http://www.geoba.se/populationphp?pc=world&page=1&type=015&st=rank&asde=&year=2044

14 https://www.ssa.gov/planners/credits.html

15 https://www.ssa.gov/planners/retire/whileworking.html

16 https://www.disability-benefits-help.org/glossary/work-credits

17 You would receive a margin call from a broker if one or more of the securities you had bought (with borrowed money) decreased in value past a certain point. You would be forced either to deposit more money in the account or to sell off some of your assets.

18 Indexed annuities are insurance contracts that, depending on the contract, may offer a guaranteed annual interest rate and some participation growth, if any, of a stock market index. Such contracts have substantial variation in terms, costs of guarantees, and features, and may cap participation or returns in significant ways. Any guarantees offered are backed by the financial strength of the insurance company. Surrender charges apply if not held to the end of the term. Withdrawals are taxed as ordinary income and, if taken prior to age fifty-nine and a half, a 10 percent federal tax penalty. Investors are cautioned to carefully review an indexed annuity for its features, costs, risks, and how the variables are calculated.

19 The National Organization of Life and Health Insurance Guaranty Associations (often abbreviated NOLHGA) is a US association made up of the life and health insurance guaranty associations of all fifty states and the District of Columbia.

20 There are two basic types of options: puts and calls. Those who own a "put" option make a profit when the market goes down, whereas those that own a "call" option profit when the market goes up.

21 The investment return and principal value of the variable annuity investment options are not guaranteed. Variable annuity sub-accounts fluctuate with changes in market conditions. The principal may be worth more or less than the original amount invested when the annuity is surrendered.

22 Variable annuities are typically invested into stocks, bonds, money market instruments, or even a combination of the three.

23 "How to Plan for Rising Health Care Costs." Edited by Fidelity, How Mutual Funds, ETFs, and Stocks Trade - Fidelity, 18 Apr. 2018, www.fidelity.com/viewpoints/personal-finance/plan-for-rising-health-care-costs.

24 https://www.seniorliving.org/lifestyles/nursing-homes/costs/

25 To qualify for some states' Medicaid programs, you must meet eligibility requirements, including income and asset limits. Income and asset limits are fixed, but if you have very high medical expenses, you may still qualify for Medicaid. This is because of a process called "spend-down" that lets you reduce or "spend down" your excess income to bring it under the "medically needy income limit." The spend-down process uses medical bills as income deductions. Medical bills are subtracted from income, and if medical bills exceed the income above the medically needy income limit, you are eligible for Medicaid, and Medicaid covers any further medical expenses.

26 https://www.irs.gov/pub/irs-pdf/i1040gi.pdf

27 https://www.irs.gov/businesses/small-businesses-self-employed/estate-tax

28 https://www.irs.gov/retirement-plans/plan-participant-employee/retirement-topics-ira-contribution-limits

29 Thorne, Deborah and Foohey, Pamela and Lawless, Robert M. and Porter, Katherine M., "Graying of U.S. Bankruptcy: Fallout from Life in a Risk Society" (August 5, 2018). Indiana Legal Studies Research Paper No. 406. Available at SSRN: https://ssrn.com/abstract=3226574 or http://dx.doi.org/10.2139/ssrn.3226574

30 Michael Finke https://www.nytimes.com/2013/05/15/business/retirementspecial/the-4-rule-for-retirement-withdrawals-may-be-outdated.html

ON CALL

EMERGENCY ROOM STORIES

VOLUME 2

DAVID BERG, M.D.

FREE REIGN

FREE REIGN
Publishing

CONTENTS

Introduction v

Chapter 1 1
Electrocution

Chapter 2 9
Stroke

Chapter 3 15
Bowel Obstruction

Chapter 4 21
Surprise Pregnancy

Chapter 5 27
Stab Wound

Chapter 6 35
Alcohol Poisoning

Chapter 7 43
Food Poisoning

Chapter 8 49
Drowning

Chapter 9 57
Hand Amputation

Chapter 10 65
Shot With An Arrow

Chapter 11 71
Missing Kidney

Publisher's Excerpt 77

Chapter 12 83
Hit and Run

Chapter 13 91
Snake Bite

Chapter 14   97
Covid

Chapter 15   105
Severe Burns

Chapter 16   113
Systemic Infection

Chapter 17   119
Spider Bite

Chapter 18   125
Allergic Reaction

Chapter 19   131
Chemical Exposure

Chapter 20   137
DVT

Chapter 21   143
Run Over

Chapter 22   149
Severe Preeclampsia

About the Author   157
Also by David Berg, M.D.   159
Also by Free Reign Publishing   161

INTRODUCTION

Welcome to my new series, *On Call: Emergency Room Stories*. As a physician who has spent countless hours in the chaotic, unpredictable world of the emergency room, I have witnessed some of the most extraordinary and unforgettable moments of my career.

In my previous series, *Stat: Crazy Medical Stories* and *Crash: Stories From the Emergency Room*, I shared with you the thrilling, heart-wrenching, and often bizarre cases that make the ER such a unique environment. From miraculous recoveries to puzzling mysteries, from heartwarming moments to sheer madness, those stories captured the essence of what it means to be on the front lines of medical care.

With *On Call*, I will take you behind the scenes, providing a raw, unfiltered look at the challenges and

triumphs we face every day. Each case is a testament to the resilience, compassion, and ingenuity of the medical professionals who dedicate their lives to saving others.

Through these stories, you'll meet patients whose courage in the face of adversity will inspire you, and you'll gain a greater appreciation for the critical role that emergency medicine plays in our healthcare system. Whether you're a seasoned medical professional, an aspiring healthcare worker, or simply someone fascinated by the drama of the ER, *On Call* offers a front-row seat to the extraordinary world of emergency medicine.

So, sit back, turn the page, and prepare to be immersed in the riveting world of the ER, where every second counts and every decision can mean the difference between life and death.

Thank you for joining me on this journey.

Sincerely,

David Berg, M.D.

CHAPTER ONE
ELECTROCUTION

The shift had started as a typical day in the emergency room, but it soon took an unexpected turn. Midway through the day, the paramedics rushed in with a patient who had suffered a severe electrical injury while working on a construction site. The patient was a middle-aged man, approximately in his mid-forties, with a robust build that indicated years of manual labor. His colleagues reported that he had been working on a high-voltage power line when the incident occurred.

Upon arrival, the patient was unresponsive, and his vital signs were unstable. His heart rate was erratic, fluctuating between bradycardia and tachycardia, with a blood pressure reading of 80/50 mmHg. His respiratory rate was shallow and labored, at 8 breaths per

minute, and his oxygen saturation was critically low at 85%. There were visible entry and exit wounds, typical of electrical burns, on his right hand and left foot.

I immediately called for the trauma team and initiated the advanced cardiac life support (ACLS) protocol. We secured the patient's airway with rapid sequence intubation to ensure adequate oxygenation. A 16-gauge intravenous line was established in the left antecubital fossa to administer fluids and medications rapidly. The patient was connected to a cardiac monitor to continuously track his heart rhythm.

The first step was to stabilize the patient's cardiovascular status. We administered an initial bolus of normal saline to combat hypotension and support circulation. Simultaneously, we began a continuous infusion of norepinephrine to maintain adequate blood pressure and perfusion. The patient's electrocardiogram (ECG) showed frequent premature ventricular contractions (PVCs) and runs of ventricular tachycardia, indicating significant cardiac instability.

Given the severity of the electrical injury, we prepared for the possibility of cardiac arrest. Calcium gluconate and sodium bicarbonate were kept ready to counteract potential electrolyte imbalances. We also administered magnesium sulfate to manage the PVCs and reduce the risk of further arrhythmias.

Attention then turned to assessing the extent of the burns and potential internal injuries. The entry wound on the right hand showed deep tissue damage with charring, indicating third-degree burns. The exit wound on the left foot was similarly severe. Both wounds were irrigated with sterile saline, and we applied dry, sterile dressings to prevent infection.

Given the high voltage involved in the injury, I was concerned about rhabdomyolysis, a condition where damaged muscle tissue releases proteins and electrolytes into the bloodstream, potentially leading to kidney failure. We initiated aggressive intravenous hydration with lactated Ringer's solution to maintain urine output and prevent myoglobin-induced renal damage. Urine output was closely monitored, aiming for at least 100 mL per hour.

To further evaluate the extent of internal damage, a portable chest X-ray and a computed tomography (CT) scan of the head, neck, chest, abdomen, and pelvis were ordered. The chest X-ray revealed no immediate signs of pneumothorax or pulmonary edema, but the CT scans showed signs of blunt force trauma to the abdomen, likely from the fall following the electrical shock. There was evidence of liver contusion and minor splenic lacerations.

Given the multi-system trauma, a multidisciplinary

approach was necessary. I consulted with the general surgery team for the abdominal injuries, the burn unit for the management of the severe burns, and the nephrology team for potential renal complications. The patient required transfer to the intensive care unit (ICU) for continuous monitoring and advanced care.

In the ICU, the treatment plan involved several critical components. Continuous ECG monitoring was essential to detect and manage arrhythmias. The patient received a regimen of intravenous fluids, including normal saline and lactated Ringer's solution, to ensure adequate hydration and support renal function. Electrolyte levels were closely monitored, with particular attention to potassium, calcium, and magnesium.

For pain management, intravenous fentanyl was administered due to its rapid onset and short duration of action, allowing for better titration. Given the risk of infection from the burns, broad-spectrum antibiotics, including vancomycin and piperacillin-tazobactam, were started empirically while awaiting culture results.

The nephrology team initiated continuous renal replacement therapy (CRRT) due to the high risk of acute kidney injury from rhabdomyolysis. This approach allowed for continuous removal of toxins and stabilization of electrolyte imbalances.

The surgical team decided against immediate exploratory laparotomy for the abdominal injuries, opting instead for serial abdominal exams and repeat imaging to monitor the liver contusion and splenic lacerations. They advised conservative management unless the patient showed signs of hemodynamic instability or worsening abdominal pain.

The burn team began the process of debridement and escharotomy for the severe electrical burns. This procedure was necessary to remove necrotic tissue and relieve the pressure from the circumferential burn wounds, which could compromise circulation and lead to compartment syndrome. Plans were made for serial wound debridements and potential skin grafting once the patient was more stable.

Throughout the night, the patient remained critically ill but stable. Continuous monitoring and aggressive supportive care were paramount. By the next morning, his condition had shown slight improvement. Blood pressure had stabilized with the help of norepinephrine, and urine output was adequate, indicating that renal function was preserved. However, his neurological status remained a concern, as he had not yet regained consciousness despite optimal oxygenation and perfusion.

A repeat CT scan of the head was performed to rule

out any delayed onset brain injury. The scan showed no acute intracranial pathology, but the patient's Glasgow Coma Scale (GCS) score remained low, indicating severe neurological impairment. An electroencephalogram (EEG) was ordered to assess brain activity and potential seizures.

Over the next few days, the patient's condition remained critical but stable. He required multiple interventions, including ongoing CRRT for renal support, repeat debridements by the burn team, and careful management of electrolytes and fluids. His cardiac status was closely monitored, with occasional episodes of ventricular tachycardia managed with amiodarone and lidocaine infusions.

By the end of the first week, the patient's renal function began to improve, allowing for the weaning off CRRT. His cardiac rhythm stabilized, and he no longer required continuous vasopressor support. However, his neurological status remained unchanged, and the prognosis for significant recovery was grim.

The patient was transferred to a specialized burn and trauma center for further management, including advanced wound care and potential reconstructive surgery. Despite the initial aggressive treatment and stabilization efforts, his overall prognosis remained

poor due to the extensive electrical injuries and associated complications.

The patient's journey through the emergency room and ICU was marked by critical interventions aimed at stabilizing his life-threatening condition. The severity of the electrical injury resulted in multi-system trauma, requiring a comprehensive and multidisciplinary approach to care. Despite the best efforts of the emergency and ICU teams, the long-term outcome remained uncertain, with significant concerns about neurological recovery and quality of life.

CHAPTER TWO
STROKE

The day began like any other in the emergency room, with the usual hustle and bustle of patients presenting with a variety of ailments. It was mid-morning when the patient arrived. The paramedics wheeled in a middle-aged man on a stretcher, his face twisted in an unnatural way. His right arm and leg were limp, and there was a pronounced droop to the right side of his face. The paramedics quickly relayed the essential details: sudden onset of symptoms, slurred speech, and weakness on the right side of the body, all classic signs of a stroke.

Time is critical in stroke cases. The window for administering life-saving treatments is narrow. As the patient was transferred from the stretcher to the ER bed, I conducted a rapid assessment. The patient's

Glasgow Coma Scale score was 11, indicating moderate impairment of consciousness. His blood pressure was elevated at 180/110 mmHg, his pulse was regular but slightly elevated, and he was afebrile. His oxygen saturation was 96% on room air.

We immediately activated the stroke protocol. A CT scan of the head without contrast was ordered to rule out hemorrhagic stroke. As we waited for the imaging results, I conducted a more detailed neurological examination. The patient's pupils were equal and reactive to light, but there was a pronounced right-sided facial droop. He exhibited profound weakness in the right upper and lower extremities, scoring 2/5 on the Medical Research Council (MRC) scale for muscle strength. His speech was garbled, and he had difficulty articulating words, a condition known as dysarthria. He also struggled to comprehend simple commands, indicating receptive aphasia.

The CT scan returned within minutes, confirming the absence of a hemorrhage. This indicated an ischemic stroke, where a clot obstructs blood flow to a part of the brain. Given the time of onset was less than four hours ago, the patient was a candidate for thrombolytic therapy. We prepared to administer tissue plasminogen activator (tPA), a clot-busting drug.

Before proceeding with tPA, we reviewed

contraindications: no recent surgeries, no history of bleeding disorders, and no evidence of gastrointestinal or urinary tract bleeding. The patient's family history and medication list were reviewed quickly to ensure no antiplatelet or anticoagulant medications had been taken. With all criteria met, we proceeded with the infusion of tPA at a dose of 0.9 mg/kg, with 10% of the total dose given as an initial bolus over one minute and the remaining 90% infused over 60 minutes.

While the tPA was administered, continuous monitoring was essential. We watched for signs of hemorrhagic transformation, a potential complication of thrombolysis. Blood pressure was closely monitored, and antihypertensive medications were ready should it exceed the safety threshold of 185/110 mmHg. The patient's neurological status was reassessed every 15 minutes during the infusion and every 30 minutes for the next six hours.

During this time, I consulted with the neurologist on call. Given the severity of the stroke, we discussed the potential need for mechanical thrombectomy if the patient did not show significant improvement after tPA administration. This procedure involves physically removing the clot using a catheter inserted through the groin and navigated to the brain's blocked artery.

After the tPA infusion, the patient's condition was

reassessed. His speech showed slight improvement, and there was a marginal increase in strength in his right arm and leg, but the deficits were still profound. It was decided to proceed with an MRI and MR angiography to assess the extent of brain injury and locate the clot precisely. The imaging revealed an occlusion in the left middle cerebral artery (MCA), confirming a significant ischemic stroke in the territory supplied by this artery.

The patient was then transferred to the interventional radiology suite for a mechanical thrombectomy. Under local anesthesia and sedation, a catheter was inserted through the femoral artery and navigated to the site of the clot. Using a stent retriever, the clot was successfully removed, restoring blood flow to the affected area of the brain.

Post-procedure, the patient was monitored in the neuro-intensive care unit (NICU). Neurological assessments continued every hour for the first 24 hours. The patient was started on a regimen of aspirin 325 mg daily to prevent further clot formation. Additionally, statin therapy with atorvastatin 80 mg daily was initiated to manage hyperlipidemia, a common risk factor for stroke. Blood pressure was managed with intravenous labetalol initially, transitioning to oral antihypertensives once the patient was stable.

Over the next 24 hours, the patient's condition

showed gradual improvement. His speech became clearer, and there was a noticeable increase in strength on his right side, though he still required assistance for basic tasks. Physical therapy, occupational therapy, and speech therapy were initiated to aid in his recovery.

As the critical period passed, the patient was reassessed by the multidisciplinary stroke team. Given his progress and potential for further recovery, a comprehensive rehabilitation plan was formulated. He was transferred to a specialized stroke rehabilitation unit where intensive therapy would continue.

The patient's hospital course was not without complications. On the third day post-stroke, he developed aspiration pneumonia, a common risk in patients with dysphagia. This was promptly treated with broad-spectrum antibiotics, and a nasogastric tube was placed for feeding to prevent further aspiration.

In the weeks that followed, the patient's condition continued to improve with rehabilitation. By the time of discharge, he had regained significant function. He was able to walk with the assistance of a cane and perform daily activities with minimal help. His speech, while still slightly slurred, had improved to the point where he could communicate effectively.

The patient was discharged on a regimen that included aspirin 81 mg daily for antiplatelet therapy,

atorvastatin 80 mg daily for lipid management, and an antihypertensive regimen tailored to his needs. Follow-up appointments with neurology, cardiology, and primary care were scheduled to ensure ongoing management of his risk factors and monitor for any signs of recurrent stroke.

While the patient's journey was far from over, and he would need ongoing rehabilitation and medical management, the prompt and coordinated efforts in the emergency room had given him the best possible chance for recovery. It was a testament to the advances in stroke care and the critical importance of time in treating this devastating condition.

CHAPTER THREE
BOWEL OBSTRUCTION

The emergency room was bustling with activity, as it always was on a Friday night. The triage nurse flagged me down, informing me of a new patient who had just arrived. I made my way through the maze of gurneys and bustling medical staff to reach the patient's room.

The patient was a middle-aged male, lying on the gurney in obvious distress. He clutched his abdomen, his face contorted in pain. His vital signs were concerning: his heart rate was elevated at 110 beats per minute, his blood pressure was low at 90/60 mmHg, and his respiratory rate was increased to 24 breaths per minute. He appeared diaphoretic and pale. The nurse handed me his initial assessment notes which indicated he had been experiencing severe abdominal pain, nausea, and vomiting for the past 24 hours.

I began my assessment with a detailed history. The patient reported that the pain started suddenly and had been progressively worsening. He had vomited multiple times, and the vomit was bilious, indicating a possible obstruction. He hadn't had a bowel movement for the past two days, and his abdomen was distended. He had a history of abdominal surgeries, which raised my suspicion for adhesions as a potential cause.

On physical examination, his abdomen was markedly distended and tympanic to percussion, with high-pitched bowel sounds, which suggested a mechanical bowel obstruction. Palpation revealed diffuse tenderness with guarding, but there was no rebound tenderness, which was somewhat reassuring against a perforation.

Given the clinical presentation, I ordered a set of labs and imaging studies. Blood work, including a complete blood count (CBC), comprehensive metabolic panel (CMP), lactate level, and arterial blood gas (ABG), was sent to the lab. I also ordered an abdominal X-ray and a CT scan with contrast of the abdomen and pelvis to further evaluate the obstruction.

While waiting for the results, I initiated intravenous access and started the patient on fluids to correct his dehydration and electrolyte imbalances. I administered 1 liter of normal saline bolus followed by maintenance

fluids. The nurse placed a nasogastric tube to decompress the stomach and relieve some of the pressure from the obstruction. The patient was also given analgesics to manage his pain and antiemetics to control his nausea and vomiting.

The X-ray showed dilated loops of bowel with air-fluid levels, consistent with a bowel obstruction. The CT scan provided a more detailed view, revealing a transition point in the small intestine with proximal dilation and distal collapse, highly suggestive of an adhesive small bowel obstruction. There were no signs of bowel ischemia or perforation on the CT scan, which was a positive sign.

The laboratory results came back, showing an elevated white blood cell count of 14,000/μL, indicative of a possible inflammatory response. His lactate level was within normal limits, which was reassuring that there was no significant tissue ischemia yet.

With the diagnosis of small bowel obstruction confirmed, I discussed the case with the on-call general surgeon. Given the patient's clinical stability and the lack of signs of strangulation or ischemia, the initial management would be non-operative. The plan was to continue with conservative management, including bowel rest, nasogastric decompression, IV fluids, and close monitoring.

The patient was admitted to the surgical floor for further observation and management. Over the next 24 hours, his condition was closely monitored. Serial abdominal exams were performed to watch for any signs of worsening or complications. His fluid status and electrolytes were meticulously managed to prevent any imbalances. Despite the initial measures, his abdominal pain persisted, and there was no significant decrease in the distension or improvement in his symptoms.

After 48 hours of conservative management without any significant improvement, the surgical team decided to take the patient to the operating room for an exploratory laparotomy. The decision was based on the lack of clinical improvement and the persistent pain, which raised concerns about potential complications that might not be apparent on imaging.

In the operating room, the surgical team found dense adhesions causing a mechanical obstruction in the small intestine. The adhesions were lysed, relieving the obstruction. The bowel appeared healthy, with no signs of necrosis or perforation. The surgery was successful, and the patient was transferred to the surgical intensive care unit for postoperative care.

In the ICU, the patient was closely monitored for any signs of postoperative complications such as infec-

tion, anastomotic leak, or further obstruction. He was kept NPO (nothing by mouth) initially, with gradual reintroduction of clear liquids as bowel function returned. Pain was managed with intravenous analgesics, and he received prophylactic antibiotics to prevent infection.

Over the next few days, the patient's condition gradually improved. His bowel sounds returned, and he started passing flatus, indicating the resolution of the obstruction. His diet was slowly advanced from clear liquids to a regular diet as tolerated. His pain decreased, and he became more comfortable.

On the fifth postoperative day, the patient was stable enough to be transferred to the regular surgical floor. He continued to show signs of improvement with normal bowel function and adequate pain control on oral medications. His electrolytes remained stable, and his surgical incision was healing well without signs of infection.

By the seventh postoperative day, the patient was ready for discharge. He was given detailed discharge instructions, including wound care, signs of potential complications to watch for, and a follow-up appointment with the surgical team. He was prescribed oral analgesics for pain management and advised to gradually return to normal activities as tolerated.

The patient left the hospital in stable condition, with a plan for outpatient follow-up to monitor his recovery and ensure no recurrence of the obstruction. His case was a reminder of the importance of timely diagnosis and intervention in managing bowel obstructions and the role of both conservative and surgical treatments in achieving a successful outcome.

The postoperative course was uneventful, leading to a successful recovery and discharge.

CHAPTER FOUR
SURPRISE PREGNANCY

The night had started as usual in the emergency room, a relentless flow of patients with various ailments and injuries. Around midnight, a patient arrived, transported by ambulance, described as an obese woman in her late thirties experiencing severe abdominal pain and shortness of breath. She was brought in on a stretcher, and I could see she was in significant distress, clutching her abdomen and gasping for air.

Upon initial examination, the patient appeared to be in obvious pain, with her vital signs showing elevated heart rate (tachycardia) and high blood pressure (hypertension). Her oxygen saturation was slightly below normal, but not alarming. Given her obesity and the nonspecific nature of her symptoms, the differential diagnosis was broad. Potential causes ranged from

gastrointestinal issues such as gallstones or pancreatitis to more severe possibilities like a myocardial infarction or a pulmonary embolism.

The first step was to get a detailed history and conduct a physical examination. The patient reported that the pain had started suddenly a few hours earlier and had progressively worsened. She also mentioned feeling nauseated but had not vomited. Her past medical history included obesity, hypertension, and type 2 diabetes, all of which could complicate her current condition.

On physical examination, the patient's abdomen was distended and tender, particularly in the lower quadrants. There were no signs of rebound tenderness or guarding, which somewhat reduced the likelihood of acute peritonitis. However, her obesity made the physical examination challenging, and I knew imaging would be crucial.

We ordered a series of blood tests, including a complete blood count (CBC), liver function tests (LFTs), amylase, lipase, and a metabolic panel. Additionally, given her shortness of breath, an electrocardiogram (ECG) and chest X-ray were performed to rule out cardiac causes and any potential respiratory issues.

While waiting for the results, I instructed the nursing staff to administer intravenous fluids to address

potential dehydration and pain relief with an opioid analgesic. Given her history of diabetes, her blood glucose levels were monitored closely, and an insulin sliding scale was initiated to manage any hyper-glycemia.

The blood tests came back with some notable find-ings. Her white blood cell count was elevated, indi-cating a possible infection or inflammatory process. Her liver enzymes were slightly elevated, but her amylase and lipase levels were within normal limits, making pancreatitis less likely. The ECG was normal, ruling out an acute myocardial infarction, and the chest X-ray showed no signs of pneumonia or other acute abnor-malities.

Given the ongoing abdominal pain and the need for further evaluation, a computed tomography (CT) scan of the abdomen and pelvis was ordered. The CT scan revealed a surprising finding: the patient had a signifi-cant amount of free fluid in the abdominal cavity and what appeared to be a large intra-abdominal mass. Additionally, there was evidence of bowel distension, suggesting a possible bowel obstruction.

At this point, the situation was becoming more urgent. The presence of free fluid raised the concern for a perforated viscus or another serious intra-abdominal pathology. The mass was an unexpected finding, and its

nature was unclear. It could be anything from an ovarian cyst to a more sinister pathology like a tumor. Given the complexity of her presentation and the need for further surgical evaluation, a consultation with the on-call surgical team was requested.

The surgical team arrived promptly and reviewed the CT findings. They concurred with the need for immediate surgical intervention to explore the cause of the free fluid and address the possible bowel obstruction. The patient was prepped for surgery, and informed consent was obtained, explaining the risks and benefits of the procedure.

During the surgery, the surgeons made a startling discovery. The mass seen on the CT scan was not a tumor or cyst, but a near-term pregnancy. The patient had been unaware of her pregnancy, likely due to her obesity masking the physical signs. The free fluid in her abdomen was due to a rupture of the amniotic sac, and the bowel obstruction was secondary to the enlarged uterus pressing against the intestines.

The surgical team quickly shifted focus to an emergency cesarean section. The baby was delivered with some difficulty due to the circumstances but was found to be alive, though in distress. Neonatal specialists were called in to assist with the immediate care of the newborn. The patient had significant internal bleeding,

likely from a uterine rupture, a life-threatening condition. The surgeons worked meticulously to control the bleeding and repair the uterus.

After what felt like an eternity, the patient was stabilized. She was transferred to the intensive care unit (ICU) for close monitoring post-surgery. The newborn was taken to the neonatal ICU for further evaluation and care. The patient's prognosis was guarded but hopeful, given the swift surgical intervention.

In the ICU, the patient was placed on a ventilator to support her breathing, and various medications were administered to manage her blood pressure and prevent infections. Broad-spectrum antibiotics were started to address any potential infection from the intra-abdominal free fluid. Blood transfusions were given to replace the significant blood loss she had suffered.

Over the next several days, the patient showed signs of gradual improvement. Her vital signs stabilized, and she was weaned off the ventilator. Her blood pressure and blood sugar levels were managed with medication, and her surgical wounds showed no signs of infection. The newborn also showed signs of improvement, though the situation remained delicate due to the premature and stressful delivery.

The patient was eventually transferred out of the ICU to a regular ward for continued recovery. Her long-

term prognosis included close follow-up with her primary care physician and specialists to manage her chronic conditions and the aftermath of her emergency surgery.

In conclusion, the case was a stark reminder of the complexities and surprises that can arise in the emergency room. The patient's initial presentation with abdominal pain and shortness of breath had led to a diagnosis of a surprise pregnancy with complications. The multidisciplinary efforts, swift surgical intervention, and intensive post-operative care were crucial in saving both the patient and her newborn. This case highlighted the importance of considering a wide differential diagnosis, especially in patients with complex medical histories and atypical presentations.

CHAPTER FIVE
STAB WOUND

The emergency room was bustling with the usual chaos when the patient arrived. It was mid-shift, and the steady stream of cases kept the team on their toes. The patient's arrival was announced by the blaring siren of the ambulance and the hurried voices of the paramedics. He was brought in on a stretcher, conscious but clearly in distress. The paramedics provided a quick rundown of the situation: the patient had sustained a stab wound to the abdomen, inflicted during an altercation.

Upon initial assessment, the patient appeared to be in his mid-thirties, with a pale complexion indicative of significant blood loss. He was sweating profusely and exhibited signs of hypovolemic shock—rapid, shallow breathing, a weak pulse, and cold, clammy skin. The

paramedics had applied a pressure dressing to the wound, but blood continued to seep through.

My first priority was to stabilize the patient. I ordered the nurse to initiate two large-bore IV lines for rapid fluid resuscitation with normal saline. Concurrently, we obtained vital signs: his blood pressure was dangerously low at 80/50 mmHg, heart rate elevated at 120 beats per minute, respiratory rate 28 breaths per minute, and oxygen saturation at 92% on room air.

The patient was clearly in pain, moaning softly and clutching his abdomen. I quickly conducted a focused assessment. The wound was located in the left upper quadrant of the abdomen, about an inch lateral to the umbilicus. The pressure dressing was already saturated with blood, and the surrounding skin was discolored, a mixture of purple and blue hues suggestive of internal bleeding.

With the immediate resuscitation measures underway, I called for a full trauma panel, including a complete blood count (CBC), comprehensive metabolic panel (CMP), coagulation profile, and type and cross-match for potential blood transfusion. Additionally, I ordered a portable chest and abdominal X-ray to assess for any potential pneumothorax or hemoperitoneum.

The patient's initial labs returned quickly. His hemoglobin was critically low at 7.2 g/dL, indicating

significant blood loss. His lactate level was elevated, a marker for poor tissue perfusion. Coagulation studies showed a slightly prolonged prothrombin time (PT) and international normalized ratio (INR), likely due to the ongoing blood loss and dilution from the IV fluids.

The X-rays showed no evidence of pneumothorax, but the abdominal film revealed free air under the diaphragm, suggesting a perforated hollow viscus. This finding, along with the clinical presentation, necessitated immediate surgical intervention.

I called for the on-call trauma surgeon and prepped the patient for transfer to the operating room. As we prepared, I inserted a Foley catheter to monitor urine output—a critical indicator of renal perfusion and overall volume status. We continued aggressive fluid resuscitation and started the patient on broad-spectrum antibiotics, given the high risk of intra-abdominal infection from a perforated bowel. Ceftriaxone and metronidazole were chosen to cover a broad range of potential pathogens.

In the interim, I performed a focused assessment with sonography for trauma (FAST) to evaluate for free fluid in the abdomen. The ultrasound confirmed the presence of significant intra-abdominal fluid, consistent with hemoperitoneum.

The trauma surgeon arrived promptly, and we

discussed the plan. Given the hemodynamic instability and the findings of the perforated viscus, the patient needed emergent exploratory laparotomy. We transferred him to the operating room, where I assisted with the transition of care.

During surgery, the extent of the damage became clear. The stab wound had penetrated the stomach and nicked the spleen, causing both active bleeding and gastrointestinal spillage into the peritoneal cavity. The surgeon worked swiftly to control the bleeding, repair the stomach laceration, and perform a splenectomy. Multiple units of packed red blood cells were transfused intraoperatively to replace the significant blood loss.

Postoperatively, the patient was transferred to the intensive care unit (ICU) for close monitoring and further management. He remained intubated and on mechanical ventilation due to his unstable condition and the need for continued sedation and pain control. We continued aggressive fluid resuscitation and blood product replacement as needed, monitoring his hemoglobin and hemodynamic status closely.

In the ICU, we implemented a comprehensive treatment plan. The patient was placed on a ventilator with settings adjusted to ensure adequate oxygenation and ventilation. We continued broad-spectrum antibiotics, initially with ceftriaxone and metronidazole, then later

de-escalated based on culture results. Pain management was critical; we administered a continuous infusion of fentanyl, titrating to effect, and supplemented with intermittent doses of midazolam for sedation.

Monitoring included continuous cardiac telemetry, hourly urine output measurements, and frequent arterial blood gas analysis to guide ventilatory support. Daily labs included a CBC, CMP, and coagulation profile to monitor for trends in blood counts, electrolytes, and liver function, which could indicate ongoing issues or complications.

On the second postoperative day, the patient's condition began to stabilize. His blood pressure normalized with the support of norepinephrine, which we were able to wean off gradually. His hemoglobin stabilized with the continued transfusion of blood products as needed, and his lactate levels trended downwards, indicating improved perfusion.

By the fourth day, the patient was alert and able to follow commands, which allowed us to assess his neurological status more thoroughly. We began the process of weaning him off the ventilator, performing spontaneous breathing trials to evaluate his readiness for extubation. His abdominal drain output decreased significantly, and repeat imaging showed no evidence of residual abscess or ongoing bleeding.

After successful extubation on the fifth day, the patient was transitioned to high-flow nasal cannula oxygen therapy and continued to receive close monitoring. His pain was managed with a combination of oral opioids and non-steroidal anti-inflammatory drugs (NSAIDs), gradually tapering the medications as his condition improved.

Throughout his ICU stay, the patient was supported by a multidisciplinary team, including intensivists, trauma surgeons, nurses, physical therapists, and nutritionists. This comprehensive approach was essential in addressing the multiple facets of his recovery, from managing his acute injuries to preventing complications such as deep vein thrombosis, pressure ulcers, and infection.

By the seventh day, the patient's condition had improved sufficiently to transfer him to the surgical ward. His diet was advanced as tolerated, starting with clear liquids and progressing to a soft diet. Physical therapy sessions focused on regaining strength and mobility, emphasizing the importance of early mobilization to reduce the risk of complications like pneumonia and muscle atrophy.

During his stay on the surgical ward, we continued to monitor his progress closely. His wound care regimen included daily dressing changes and the application of

topical antibiotics to prevent infection. His pain was managed effectively with oral medications, and his overall condition continued to improve.

The patient was discharged home after two weeks in the hospital, with detailed discharge instructions and a follow-up plan. He was prescribed a course of oral antibiotics to complete, along with pain medications to manage any residual discomfort. We provided instructions for wound care, signs of infection to watch for, and scheduled follow-up appointments with both the trauma surgeon and his primary care physician to ensure continuity of care.

In the follow-up visits, the patient showed remarkable improvement. His surgical wounds were healing well, and there were no signs of infection or complications. His hemoglobin levels had normalized, and he reported a gradual return to his usual activities, although with some residual fatigue and weakness, which was expected given the severity of his injuries and the recovery process.

CHAPTER SIX
ALCOHOL POISONING

When the patient was wheeled into the emergency room, it was clear that this would be a challenging case. A young college student, around 19 or 20 years old, had been found unconscious at a fraternity party. According to the brief report from the paramedics, he had been drinking heavily throughout the night. The patient had consumed an unknown quantity of alcohol in a short period, which led to his current critical condition. His friends had called 911 when they noticed he was unresponsive and not breathing normally.

The first assessment in the emergency room revealed a deeply concerning situation. The patient's skin was pale and clammy, and he had a very slow and irregular pulse. His respiratory rate was dangerously low, and he exhibited a Glasgow Coma Scale (GCS)

score of 6, indicating severe impairment of consciousness. The smell of alcohol was potent, even from a
distance. His blood pressure was dangerously low at
80/50 mmHg. Immediate intervention was crucial to
prevent further deterioration.

I ordered a rapid sequence of actions to stabilize the
patient. Firstly, we ensured his airway was secure.
Given his compromised level of consciousness and the
risk of aspiration, intubation was necessary. A skilled
anesthesiologist inserted the endotracheal tube while I
prepared for the next steps. Once intubated, we initiated mechanical ventilation to maintain adequate
oxygenation and ventilation.

Intravenous access was quickly established with
two large-bore IV lines. I ordered a bolus of normal
saline to address his hypotension, followed by a continuous infusion to maintain adequate blood pressure. The
initial blood work included a complete blood count
(CBC), basic metabolic panel (BMP), liver function tests
(LFTs), and, crucially, a blood alcohol concentration
(BAC) test.

The blood alcohol concentration results were
alarming but not unexpected. The patient's BAC was
0.38%, nearly five times the legal limit for driving and
well within the range of potentially fatal alcohol
poisoning. His electrolytes were also deranged, with

significant hypokalemia and mild hyponatremia, likely exacerbated by the excessive alcohol intake and associated dehydration.

Given the patient's severe alcohol poisoning, we initiated several critical treatments simultaneously. Thiamine was administered intravenously to prevent Wernicke's encephalopathy, a neurological disorder that can occur due to alcohol abuse. Additionally, I ordered magnesium sulfate to correct any potential deficiencies, as chronic alcohol users are often deficient in magnesium, which can contribute to cardiac arrhythmias.

To manage the hypokalemia, we started a potassium chloride infusion, carefully monitoring his potassium levels to avoid the risk of hyperkalemia. I also prescribed folic acid to address potential deficiencies and support overall recovery. Continuous cardiac monitoring was essential to detect any arrhythmias early, given his electrolyte imbalances and severe intoxication.

As we worked on stabilizing the patient, we also considered the potential for other complications. Acute alcohol poisoning can lead to hypoglycemia, so regular blood glucose checks were mandatory. Indeed, his initial blood glucose was slightly low at 65 mg/dL. We administered an IV bolus of dextrose to correct this,

followed by a glucose infusion to maintain stable blood sugar levels.

Throughout the treatment process, we monitored the patient's vital signs closely. Despite the aggressive fluid resuscitation, his blood pressure remained borderline low. I decided to initiate a vasopressor infusion, specifically norepinephrine, to support his cardiovascular system and maintain adequate perfusion to vital organs.

Once the initial stabilization measures were in place, we conducted a thorough physical examination to identify any signs of trauma or other underlying conditions that could complicate his situation. Thankfully, there were no indications of head injury, internal bleeding, or other acute physical trauma. However, his liver function tests showed elevated transaminases, suggesting possible acute alcoholic hepatitis or stress on the liver due to excessive alcohol intake.

Given the severity of his condition, it was imperative to transfer the patient to the intensive care unit (ICU) for ongoing monitoring and management. In the ICU, he would receive continuous support for his cardiovascular and respiratory systems, and his electrolyte imbalances would be managed with meticulous care.

Additionally, the ICU team could provide more advanced monitoring for potential complications such as seizures or worsening hepatic function.

Before transferring the patient, I ensured that a comprehensive handover was provided to the ICU team. This included detailing his initial presentation, the treatments administered in the emergency room, and the current management plan. We discussed the need for continued cardiac monitoring, regular blood glucose checks, and the importance of correcting his electrolyte imbalances.

As the patient was wheeled to the ICU, I felt a mix of relief and concern. We had managed to stabilize him in the emergency room, but his condition remained critical. The next 24 to 48 hours would be crucial in determining his outcome. Alcohol poisoning at such a severe level posed significant risks, including potential brain damage, cardiac complications, and liver failure.

The following morning, I checked on the patient's progress in the ICU. The initial signs were cautiously optimistic. His vital signs had stabilized somewhat, and his blood pressure was holding steady with the help of the vasopressor infusion. The electrolyte imbalances were being corrected gradually, and his blood glucose levels were within the normal range. However, he remained deeply unconscious, and the medical

team was vigilant for any signs of neurological recovery.

Over the next few days, the patient showed slow but steady improvement. The mechanical ventilation was gradually weaned as his respiratory function improved. The continuous monitoring allowed us to adjust treatments dynamically, ensuring that any fluctuations in his condition were addressed promptly. His liver function tests began to normalize, indicating that his liver was starting to recover from the acute insult of alcohol poisoning.

After five days in the ICU, the patient regained consciousness. This was a significant milestone, suggesting that despite the severity of his alcohol poisoning, he had avoided major neurological damage. His GCS score improved, and he began to respond to verbal commands. The medical team started to reduce the sedation, allowing for a clearer assessment of his cognitive functions.

As the patient became more alert, we transitioned him from the ICU to a step-down unit for continued monitoring and rehabilitation. The focus now was on supporting his recovery and addressing any lingering issues related to his alcohol use. A psychiatric evaluation was arranged to assess his mental health and provide counseling on the dangers of binge drinking.

The patient's recovery continued steadily, and after two weeks in the hospital, he was deemed stable enough for discharge. He was prescribed oral potassium supplements to maintain his electrolyte balance and a multivitamin to support his overall health. Additionally, he received a referral to an outpatient rehabilitation program to address his alcohol use and prevent future episodes of excessive drinking.

Reflecting on the case, it was clear that the rapid and coordinated efforts of the emergency room and ICU teams had been pivotal in saving the patient's life. Severe alcohol poisoning is a life-threatening condition that requires immediate and aggressive intervention. The patient's recovery was a testament to the effectiveness of evidence-based medical protocols and the dedication of the healthcare professionals involved in his care.

Despite the positive outcome, the case underscored the critical need for greater awareness and prevention efforts around alcohol abuse, particularly among college students. Education on the dangers of binge drinking and accessible support services for those struggling with alcohol use are essential in preventing such life-threatening incidents.

The patient's story could have ended tragically, but thanks to the timely medical intervention, he had a

second chance. It was a stark reminder of the fragility of life and the profound impact of alcohol on young lives. The hope was that this experience would be a turning point for the patient, leading to healthier choices and a brighter future free from the dangers of excessive drinking.

CHAPTER SEVEN
FOOD POISONING

The night shift in the emergency room had always been the most demanding. There was a relentless stream of patients, each bringing their own emergencies and stories. But nothing could have prepared me for the case that unfolded on a stormy summer night.

It began with the frantic arrival of a group of four teenagers. The first was wheeled in, pale and unresponsive, followed by the others, each in various stages of distress. My heart sank as I observed the severity of their conditions. Their symptoms were strikingly similar: profuse vomiting, severe abdominal pain, and diarrhea. The smell of vomit and fear filled the room.

The nurses quickly set to work, and I was thrust into a maelstrom of urgent decision-making. My immediate concern was stabilizing the patients. The first, a boy

about sixteen years old, was the most critical. He was unresponsive, his skin cold and clammy, his pulse weak and thready. His vital signs showed severe hypotension, tachycardia, and signs of shock. My initial assessment pointed towards severe dehydration and hypovolemic shock.

We initiated aggressive fluid resuscitation with isotonic saline. I ordered blood tests, including complete blood count, electrolytes, renal function, liver function tests, and blood cultures. We also sent samples for stool cultures and tested for common foodborne pathogens. Meanwhile, a nasogastric tube was inserted to decompress the stomach and alleviate some of the pressure.

As the fluids began to infuse, we inserted a Foley catheter to monitor urine output, an essential indicator of renal perfusion and overall fluid status. His oxygen saturation was borderline, so we administered supplemental oxygen via a non-rebreather mask to ensure adequate tissue oxygenation. While waiting for lab results, I considered the possible causes: bacterial gastroenteritis, viral infections, and food poisoning.

The other three teenagers were not faring much better. Two of them, a boy and a girl, exhibited similar symptoms, though they were still semi-conscious and able to respond to questions with difficulty. The fourth,

another girl, was in a state of severe distress but not yet unresponsive. We initiated the same protocol for them: intravenous fluids, monitoring, and broad-spectrum antibiotics while we awaited further information.

Despite our efforts, the condition of the first boy did not improve. His blood pressure remained critically low, and his heart rate continued to race. We administered vasopressors to maintain his blood pressure, starting with norepinephrine. His lab results began to trickle in, revealing profound metabolic acidosis, elevated white blood cell count, and signs of acute kidney injury. The stool cultures and blood tests were still pending.

Hours passed, and the emergency room was a hive of activity. The other three teenagers' conditions fluctuated, but none deteriorated as rapidly as the first. Unfortunately, despite all interventions, the first boy went into cardiac arrest. We performed CPR for over thirty minutes, but there was no return of spontaneous circulation. Time of death was pronounced, and the mood in the ER grew somber. One life lost.

Meanwhile, the condition of the second boy worsened. He exhibited signs of sepsis: high fever, hypotension, and altered mental status. His blood cultures eventually grew out Salmonella typhimurium, a bacterium often associated with foodborne illnesses. This finding narrowed our focus and confirmed our

suspicion of a severe foodborne infection. Broad-spec-trum antibiotics were continued, and we added targeted therapy with ciprofloxacin.

The two girls showed similar bacterial growth in their cultures. Both were switched to the same targeted antibiotic regimen. Despite our best efforts, the second boy succumbed to his illness. His septic shock was too severe, and his organs began to fail one by one. The remaining two patients were stabilized, though their conditions were still critical.

We transferred the third patient, the girl in the worst condition, to the intensive care unit. She required mechanical ventilation due to respiratory failure and continuous renal replacement therapy for her kidneys, which had stopped functioning adequately. Her prog-nosis was guarded, and we could only hope that the antibiotics would control the infection before it caused irreversible damage.

The fourth patient, although still critically ill, responded better to the treatment. Her fever started to subside, and her vital signs stabilized. She was also transferred to the ICU but did not require mechanical ventilation. The fluid resuscitation and antibiotics seemed to be taking effect, and there was a glimmer of hope in her recovery.

Days passed, and we received updates from the ICU.

The third patient fought valiantly, but her body eventually gave in to the infection and its complications. The news hit us hard; three of the four teenagers had died. It was a devastating outcome, one that lingered heavily in the minds of everyone who had been involved in their care.

The last patient, however, showed remarkable resilience. She began to recover gradually, her kidney function started to improve, and she was weaned off the ventilator. It took weeks, but she eventually stabilized enough to be moved out of the ICU and into a regular ward. Her recovery was slow but steady, and she became the sole survivor of the group.

Reflecting on the case, the diagnosis was clear: severe Salmonella typhimurium infection leading to septic shock and multi-organ failure. The treatment plan was comprehensive but ultimately insufficient to save three of the four teenagers. For the surviving patient, the combination of aggressive fluid resuscitation, broad-spectrum antibiotics followed by targeted therapy, and intensive supportive care in the ICU made the difference.

In the end, the patient who survived was discharged with a long road to full recovery ahead. She would require follow-up appointments, monitoring of her kidney function, and a gradual return to normalcy. The

loss of her friends was a heavy burden, and psychological support was arranged to help her cope with the trauma.

This case left an indelible mark on me. It was a stark reminder of the fragility of life and the relentless nature of bacterial infections. Despite the advanced medical interventions available, some battles are still lost. But it also highlighted the resilience of the human body and spirit. The patient who survived was a testament to that resilience, a beacon of hope amidst the tragedy.

As an emergency room doctor, I faced numerous challenges and heart-wrenching moments, but none quite like this. The memory of those four teenagers and the battle we fought to save them will stay with me forever, a reminder of the importance of vigilance, rapid response, and the relentless pursuit of saving lives.

CHAPTER EIGHT
DROWNING

I was nearing the end of my shift in the emergency room when the call came in. A man had fallen into a frozen lake and had to be resuscitated at the scene by emergency responders. The frigid waters had claimed his body temperature, plunging him into severe hypothermia. The paramedics managed to restore a pulse after a harrowing twenty minutes of CPR, and he was en route to our hospital.

As the paramedics wheeled him in, I immediately noted his pale, waxy skin and the lifeless appearance typical of severe hypothermia. His core temperature was recorded at 28 degrees Celsius (82.4 degrees Fahrenheit), far below the normal body temperature of 37 degrees Celsius (98.6 degrees Fahrenheit). He was

unconscious, and his vital signs were tenuous at best. His heart rate was slow and erratic, and his blood pressure was critically low.

The first order of business was to stabilize his heart rhythm and elevate his body temperature. We transferred him to a trauma bed, and I quickly ordered the initiation of active internal rewarming. A heated blanket was placed over him, and warm intravenous fluids were administered through a central line to ensure rapid and effective warming from the inside out. We also inserted a urinary catheter to monitor his core temperature more accurately.

An electrocardiogram (EKG) revealed classic signs of hypothermia, including Osborn waves, which are extra deflections following the QRS complex. These waves are often seen in severe hypothermia and indicate a heightened risk of cardiac arrhythmias. To combat this, we began a continuous infusion of warmed saline and kept a defibrillator on standby in case his heart rhythm deteriorated further.

Simultaneously, a blood gas analysis showed significant metabolic acidosis, a condition where the body produces excess acid or when the kidneys are not removing enough acid from the body. This was likely due to the prolonged period of inadequate oxygenation and circulation during the time he was submerged and

the subsequent resuscitation efforts. We administered sodium bicarbonate to counteract the acidosis and stabilize his pH levels.

Given the prolonged CPR and his current state, I suspected that the patient might also have suffered some degree of anoxic brain injury, which occurs due to lack of oxygen to the brain. To assess the extent of this injury, we ordered a head CT scan. We also checked his blood glucose levels, which were critically low, necessitating the immediate administration of dextrose.

While waiting for the results of the CT scan, I reviewed his lab work. The patient had severe electrolyte imbalances, with dangerously low potassium and magnesium levels. Both of these are crucial for proper heart function and could exacerbate his risk of arrhythmias. I ordered intravenous potassium chloride and magnesium sulfate to correct these deficiencies.

The CT scan revealed cerebral edema, a common consequence of anoxic brain injury, indicating that the patient's brain had swollen due to the lack of oxygen. To manage this, we administered mannitol, an osmotic diuretic, to reduce the swelling and prevent further brain damage. We also initiated a continuous infusion of hypertonic saline to help draw excess fluid out of the brain tissues.

Despite our best efforts, the patient's heart rate

became increasingly erratic, transitioning into ventricular fibrillation, a life-threatening heart rhythm that
results in rapid, inadequate heartbeats. We immediately
performed defibrillation, delivering a shock to his heart
to try and restore a normal rhythm. After three shocks
and a dose of intravenous epinephrine, his heart
rhythm stabilized to a slow but regular rate.

We then inserted a nasogastric tube to decompress
his stomach, which was likely filled with cold water,
contributing to his hypothermia. Aspiration of the cold
water also posed a risk of secondary drowning, where
inhaled water causes lung damage and subsequent
respiratory distress. The tube allowed us to suction out
the water and administer activated charcoal to bind any
ingested toxins that could have been in the lake water.

Next, we focused on his respiratory function. His
oxygen saturation was perilously low, and he was
exhibiting signs of acute respiratory distress syndrome
(ARDS), likely triggered by the aspiration of lake water.
We intubated him and placed him on mechanical ventilation with high levels of positive end-expiratory pressure (PEEP) to keep his alveoli open and improve
oxygen exchange.

In parallel, we initiated broad-spectrum antibiotics
to preempt any infections from potential pathogens in

the lake water. His immune system, already compromised by the severe hypothermia and prolonged resuscitation, was particularly vulnerable to sepsis.

Monitoring his kidney function was also crucial, given the possibility of acute kidney injury from rhabdomyolysis, a condition where damaged muscle tissue breaks down rapidly, releasing myoglobin into the bloodstream, which can damage the kidneys. To prevent this, we maintained high urine output with aggressive fluid resuscitation and monitored his kidney function through serial blood tests.

Over the next few hours, his core temperature slowly began to rise, and his vital signs stabilized, albeit tenuously. We continued to monitor his heart rhythm closely and adjusted his electrolyte levels as needed. His metabolic acidosis improved with the bicarbonate therapy, and his blood gas analysis showed a gradual return to normal pH levels.

Despite these improvements, the prognosis remained guarded. The cerebral edema indicated significant brain injury, and it was unclear how much neurological function he would regain, if any. We kept him sedated and continued to monitor intracranial pressure, adjusting his medications as necessary to control the swelling.

After 24 hours of intensive treatment in the emergency room, the patient was stable enough for transfer to the intensive care unit (ICU). There, he would receive continuous monitoring and specialized care to manage his complex condition. The ICU team was briefed on his case, including the details of his hypothermia treatment, electrolyte management, and ongoing concerns about his brain and kidney function.

Over the next week, the patient's condition remained critical. Despite our efforts to manage the cerebral edema, he showed minimal signs of neurological improvement. An MRI confirmed extensive brain damage, and his prognosis for meaningful recovery was bleak. His family, who had been notified and were now at his bedside, faced the difficult decision of whether to continue aggressive treatment or consider palliative care options.

Ultimately, the family decided to prioritize comfort and dignity, transitioning him to a palliative care plan. The ventilator was gradually weaned, and he was kept comfortable with analgesics and sedatives. The medical team provided compassionate support to the family, explaining each step of the process and ensuring that the patient's final days were as peaceful as possible.

The patient passed away peacefully three days later.

The tragic outcome underscored the formidable challenges of severe hypothermia and the profound impact
of prolonged oxygen deprivation on the brain. Despite
the aggressive and comprehensive efforts to save him,
the extent of his injuries was insurmountable.

CHAPTER NINE
HAND AMPUTATION

The call came in at 2:47 PM, a code red trauma alert. The patient was en route to our emergency room, a middle-aged male who had suffered a catastrophic injury at a local factory. As the on-call emergency room doctor, I mentally prepared for the worst. The brief information relayed by the paramedics indicated that the patient's right hand had been amputated by heavy machinery, and they were struggling to control the bleeding.

Upon arrival, the patient was wheeled into the trauma bay, surrounded by a flurry of paramedics and nurses. The atmosphere was charged with urgency. The patient was pale and diaphoretic, indicative of significant blood loss. His right arm was heavily bandaged, soaked through with blood, and the crude tourniquet

applied by the paramedics was the only thing keeping him from exsanguinating.

I quickly assessed the patient's vitals. His blood pressure was dangerously low at 80/40 mmHg, and his heart rate was elevated at 130 beats per minute, signs of hypovolemic shock. The paramedics reported that the amputation had occurred approximately 30 minutes prior. We had no time to lose.

The initial step was to establish two large-bore IV lines to administer fluids and blood products. I ordered 2 liters of normal saline to be infused rapidly to stabilize his blood pressure. Simultaneously, I directed the nurses to prepare for a massive transfusion protocol, anticipating the need for multiple units of packed red blood cells, fresh frozen plasma, and platelets to replace the significant blood loss.

Next, I removed the makeshift tourniquet and carefully inspected the wound. The amputation was complete, just proximal to the wrist, with jagged edges indicating a traumatic severance rather than a clean cut. The exposed tissue and bone were covered with debris and grease, requiring immediate irrigation to prevent infection.

We irrigated the wound with copious amounts of sterile saline to remove contaminants. The patient

grimaced in pain, despite the fentanyl administered by the paramedics for pain management. I ordered an additional dose of morphine for more effective pain control.

Controlling the bleeding was paramount. I applied a pneumatic tourniquet above the elbow to temporarily stop the hemorrhage while we worked. Next, I methodically clamped and ligated the severed blood vessels to prevent further blood loss. This process was painstaking, but critical for stabilizing the patient. Once the bleeding was controlled, we covered the wound with sterile dressings.

While we worked on the immediate physical stabilization, I considered the next steps in the patient's care. Given the severity of the injury and the potential for complications, I contacted the orthopedic and vascular surgeons to arrange for an emergency surgical consult. Reattachment of the hand would likely be impossible due to the nature of the injury and the elapsed time since the amputation, but a formal evaluation was necessary to determine the best course of action.

The patient's condition stabilized somewhat after the initial resuscitation efforts. His blood pressure improved to 100/60 mmHg, and his heart rate decreased to 110 beats per minute. However, he

remained at high risk for complications, including infection, further blood loss, and the potential for shock.

I ordered broad-spectrum antibiotics, specifically a combination of ceftriaxone and metronidazole, to address the risk of infection from the contaminated wound. Tetanus prophylaxis was also administered given the dirty nature of the injury.

Throughout the entire process, the patient remained conscious but in significant distress. The psychological trauma of losing a limb in such a sudden and violent manner was evident. I ensured that a member of our psychiatric team was available to provide immediate support and planned for a follow-up consultation to address the emotional and psychological aspects of his injury.

The next critical step was preparing the patient for transfer to the operating room. The orthopedic surgeon arrived and concurred with my assessment that reattachment was not feasible. The focus would instead be on debridement of the wound, securing hemostasis, and planning for a future prosthesis. The vascular surgeon was on hand to assess the need for any additional vascular repairs.

As we prepared for surgery, I reviewed the patient's lab results. His hemoglobin level was 7.2 g/dL,

confirming significant blood loss. I ordered an additional two units of packed red blood cells to be transfused. His white blood cell count was slightly elevated, likely a stress response to the trauma, but also a potential early sign of infection.

The patient was prepped and transported to the operating room, where the surgical team took over. The debridement was extensive, removing damaged tissue and ensuring that all foreign material was eliminated to minimize the risk of infection. The surgeons then fashioned a flap from the remaining tissue to cover the stump, creating a foundation for a future prosthetic fitting.

Post-operatively, the patient was transferred to the intensive care unit for close monitoring. He was placed on intravenous antibiotics and continued to receive blood products as needed to maintain his hemoglobin levels. Pain management remained a priority, and a regimen of intravenous opioids was instituted, transitioning to oral medications as his condition improved.

Over the next 48 hours, the patient's condition stabilized. His vital signs normalized, and the wound showed no immediate signs of infection. The psychological impact of the injury was profound, and he began sessions with our psychiatric team to address his acute

distress and to start the long process of psychological healing.

Three days post-injury, the patient was transferred from the ICU to a regular surgical ward. His pain was managed with a combination of opioids and non-steroidal anti-inflammatory drugs, and he was started on physical therapy to begin adapting to life with a significant disability.

In follow-up visits, the focus shifted to rehabilitation and planning for a prosthetic. The patient struggled with the loss of his dominant hand, facing challenges in performing basic tasks. Occupational therapy became a crucial part of his recovery, helping him develop new skills and coping strategies.

Six weeks after the injury, the patient returned for a final surgical follow-up. The stump had healed well without infection, and plans were made for fitting a prosthetic hand. His emotional state remained fragile, but ongoing psychiatric support and the encouragement of his family and friends provided a foundation for recovery.

The road to recovery was long and arduous. The patient faced numerous physical and emotional challenges, but with comprehensive medical and psychological support, he began to rebuild his life. The loss of a limb is a life-altering event, but through resilience and

the dedicated efforts of the entire medical team, he found a path forward.

Though the patient's journey was marked by pain and loss, it also highlighted the capacity for human resilience and the vital role of comprehensive medical care in navigating the aftermath of traumatic injuries.

CHAPTER TEN
SHOT WITH AN ARROW

The emergency room is a place where the unexpected becomes routine, where the bizarre becomes almost mundane. It was a busy Saturday afternoon when the call came in. We were alerted about a teenager en route to our facility, shot with an arrow. The details were sparse; he and a friend had been shooting arrows into the sky, and one had come back down, striking him in the shoulder. It was an unusual but not entirely unheard-of accident.

Upon arrival, the paramedics rushed the patient into the trauma bay. He was a young male, approximately 16 years old, pale and visibly in pain but conscious and alert. The arrow protruded grotesquely from his left shoulder, just below the clavicle. Blood

seeped steadily from the wound, soaking through the makeshift bandages the paramedics had applied.

The first priority was stabilizing the patient. We initiated intravenous access, starting with two large-bore IVs for fluid resuscitation, anticipating significant blood loss. Vital signs were taken immediately: heart rate elevated at 120 beats per minute, blood pressure low at 90/60 mmHg, and respiratory rate at 24 breaths per minute. The patient was clearly in distress, both from pain and hypovolemia.

Next, we needed to assess the extent of the injury. The arrow's shaft was made of wood, and it appeared to be deeply embedded. We needed imaging to determine the trajectory and to assess for any damage to vital structures. We ordered an immediate portable X-ray of the chest and shoulder. While waiting for the imaging, I conducted a focused physical exam. There was no evidence of a pneumothorax—no tracheal deviation, no asymmetrical chest expansion, and breath sounds were equal bilaterally. However, the arrow's position suggested it might have punctured the subclavian artery or vein, which could explain the ongoing blood loss.

The X-ray images arrived quickly, revealing that the arrow had indeed penetrated deeply, but miraculously, it had missed the subclavian artery by a mere centime-

ter. It had, however, nicked the subclavian vein, causing significant bleeding. Additionally, the tip of the arrow was perilously close to the apex of the lung, posing a risk of pneumothorax if not handled delicately.

Given the complexity of the situation, I decided to consult with the vascular surgery and cardiothoracic teams. We needed their expertise for the removal of the arrow and for the potential repair of the subclavian vein. Meanwhile, we continued to monitor the patient's vital signs and maintained fluid resuscitation with normal saline.

The patient's pain was becoming increasingly unmanageable despite the administration of intravenous morphine. The arrow's position made it impossible to move him without exacerbating his pain or potentially worsening his condition. We needed to act swiftly but cautiously.

The vascular surgeon arrived and reviewed the X-rays. He concurred with my assessment and outlined a plan: the arrow would be removed in the operating room under controlled conditions to prevent any sudden hemorrhage or lung injury. The patient was prepped for surgery. We administered broad-spectrum antibiotics prophylactically to prevent infection, as the wooden arrow could introduce bacteria deep into the tissue.

During the transfer to the operating room, we ensured continuous monitoring of vital signs. The anesthesiologist took over, administering general anesthesia to keep the patient sedated and pain-free during the procedure. The surgical team moved with precision, making an incision to expose the entry wound fully. The arrow was carefully extracted, millimeter by millimeter, to minimize tissue damage. As anticipated, the subclavian vein was injured, and the surgeon quickly repaired the tear using fine sutures. The lung, fortunately, remained unscathed.

Once the arrow was removed and the vein repaired, the surgical team ensured there was no ongoing bleeding. They placed a drain to prevent any accumulation of blood or fluid in the area and closed the incision. The patient was then moved to the post-anesthesia care unit (PACU) for recovery and close monitoring.

Back in the emergency department, I reviewed the case notes and updated the patient's medical record. Post-operative orders included continuation of IV fluids, pain management with morphine titrated to effect, and regular monitoring of hematocrit and hemoglobin levels to ensure there was no delayed bleeding. I also ordered a follow-up chest X-ray to rule out any secondary pneumothorax from the procedure.

As the hours passed, the patient began to stabilize.

His vital signs improved—heart rate down to 90 beats per minute, blood pressure normalized to 120/80 mmHg, and respiratory rate at a steady 18 breaths per minute. The post-operative chest X-ray showed no evidence of pneumothorax, and the drain output was minimal, indicating that the bleeding had been effectively controlled.

We transitioned the patient from intravenous morphine to oral pain medication, starting with oxycodone. Antibiotics were continued to prevent infection, initially with broad-spectrum coverage and later tailored based on culture results from the wound. The patient was also given tetanus prophylaxis, considering the nature of the injury.

The next step was ensuring the patient's smooth transition to the surgical floor for continued care. I coordinated with the surgical team and the floor nurses, providing a detailed handoff about the injury, the surgical repair, and the ongoing treatment plan. The patient was transferred with continuous monitoring, and his family was updated on his condition and prognosis.

Over the next few days, the patient's recovery progressed well. The surgical team performed regular wound checks and adjusted the antibiotic regimen as needed. Physical therapy was consulted to assist with

shoulder mobility and to prevent stiffness and loss of function. Pain management was optimized with a combination of acetaminophen and ibuprofen, reducing the need for stronger opioids.

After a week, the patient was stable enough to be discharged home with detailed instructions for wound care, signs of infection to watch for, and a follow-up appointment with the vascular surgeon. He was advised to refrain from any strenuous activities that could stress the healing tissue and to attend all scheduled physical therapy sessions.

In follow-up visits, the patient showed excellent progress. The wound healed without signs of infection, and the subclavian vein repair remained intact with no signs of thrombosis or other complications. His shoulder function gradually returned to normal with the help of physical therapy.

Reflecting on this case, the rapid response and collaboration among the emergency, surgical, and anesthesiology teams were crucial in managing a potentially fatal injury. The initial assessment and stabilization, followed by precise surgical intervention and meticulous post-operative care, ensured the patient's recovery.

Despite the unusual circumstances, the patient's outcome was favorable due to timely intervention and comprehensive care.

CHAPTER ELEVEN
MISSING KIDNEY

The call came in around midnight. I was nearing the end of my shift when the radio crackled to life with the paramedics' report. A male in his mid-thirties was found unconscious in an alley, disoriented and in obvious distress. When he woke, he reported severe abdominal pain and found himself in a pool of his own blood. The paramedics suspected foul play and rushed him to our emergency room.

When the patient arrived, he was pale, sweating profusely, and in visible agony. His vitals were alarming: blood pressure was dangerously low at 80/50 mmHg, heart rate elevated at 120 beats per minute, and his respiratory rate was rapid and shallow. The patient was also running a fever of 101°F, indicating a possible infection. He was groggy but managed to tell us he had been

given a tranquilizer by an unknown assailant and had no recollection of the events that followed until he woke up in the alley.

I began my assessment immediately. His abdomen was distended, and upon palpation, he exhibited rebound tenderness, especially in the right lower quadrant. There was also a large, hastily stitched incision on his right flank, indicating some sort of crude surgical procedure. His skin around the wound was inflamed and warm to the touch, with purulent discharge seeping from the sutures. It was evident that the patient had undergone an illicit surgery, and the suspicion was that one of his kidneys had been removed.

Given the critical nature of his condition, we initiated the standard emergency protocols. We started with securing his airway and administering oxygen to ensure he was adequately perfused. Two large-bore IV lines were established for fluid resuscitation with normal saline to combat his hypovolemic shock. We sent off blood samples for a complete blood count, electrolytes, renal function tests, blood cultures, and type and crossmatch for possible blood transfusion.

An immediate ultrasound of the abdomen confirmed our worst fears: his right kidney was indeed missing. There was free fluid in the abdomen, likely blood, suggesting internal bleeding. The remaining

kidney appeared to be functioning, but it was under significant strain, as indicated by the initial lab results showing elevated creatinine levels and a decreased glomerular filtration rate.

We prepped the patient for an emergency laparotomy to control the bleeding, debride the infected wound, and assess any further damage. Antibiotic therapy was started with broad-spectrum antibiotics—piperacillin-tazobactam and vancomycin—given the high risk of sepsis from the contaminated wound. Analgesics were administered judiciously to manage his pain without further compromising his already low blood pressure.

In the operating room, the extent of the damage became more apparent. The kidney had been removed with crude instruments, leaving behind torn blood vessels and significant internal bleeding. The surgical team worked swiftly to ligate the bleeding vessels, remove necrotic tissue, and clean the infected area. A drain was placed to allow any remaining pus and fluids to exit the body, and the incision was closed with more secure sutures.

Post-operatively, the patient was transferred to the intensive care unit for close monitoring. He remained on intravenous fluids, and we started him on a low-dose norepinephrine infusion to support his blood pressure.

His urine output was closely monitored to assess the function of his remaining kidney. Blood transfusions were given to replace the blood lost during the surgery and improve his overall hemodynamic status.

Over the next 24 hours, the patient remained in a critical but stable condition. His vital signs gradually improved, and his urine output increased, suggesting that his remaining kidney was compensating for the loss. Repeat blood tests showed a slow return towards normal renal function, though he would need long-term follow-up to monitor for chronic kidney disease.

As the days passed, the patient's condition continued to stabilize. The infection was brought under control with the continued course of antibiotics, and his fever subsided. Pain management was adjusted to oral medications as his condition improved, and he was able to tolerate a light diet.

The patient's recovery was remarkable given the severity of his initial presentation. After a week in the ICU, he was transferred to a general medical ward for further recovery and physical therapy. We involved a multidisciplinary team, including nephrologists, infectious disease specialists, and a trauma surgeon, to plan his long-term care.

Before discharge, we educated the patient on signs of potential complications, such as symptoms of infec-

tion or kidney failure, and emphasized the importance of regular follow-up appointments. He was prescribed a course of oral antibiotics to complete the treatment of the infection, as well as antihypertensive medication to manage his blood pressure, which was now under strain due to the single kidney. Pain was managed with non-opioid analgesics to avoid the risk of addiction.

We also arranged for psychological support, as the traumatic nature of his assault and the subsequent loss of a kidney could have significant mental health repercussions. The patient was encouraged to attend counseling sessions and was given information on support groups for victims of violent crime.

Upon discharge, the patient was stable, ambulating independently, and able to perform basic daily activities. He was given detailed instructions on wound care and signs of complications. A follow-up appointment was scheduled with the nephrology team to monitor his kidney function and adjust his medications as needed.

The patient's prognosis was cautiously optimistic. With only one kidney, he would need to be vigilant about maintaining a healthy lifestyle and avoiding factors that could further strain his renal function. Regular check-ups and adherence to medical advice were crucial for his long-term health.

Meningitis

It was just another ordinary shift when the call came in. A college girl, unconscious in her dorm room. The

details were sparse, as they often are. Dispatch mentioned a possible case of meningitis. I sighed, my mind already racing through the protocol. Meningitis—never a good sign. I geared up, hopped into the ambulance, and we sped off to the address.

Arriving at the dorm, I grabbed my kit and rushed inside. The dormitory was the typical chaos you'd expect from a college: loud music, students milling around, and the unmistakable smell of a thousand instant noodle cups. I navigated the narrow hallways and finally reached the room. A campus security officer stood by the door, looking more nervous than he probably should have been. I brushed past him and entered.

There she was, sprawled on her bed, looking almost peaceful if it weren't for the alarming situation. I quickly checked for a pulse and breathing. Pulse was there, albeit weak, and her breathing was shallow. Her skin was pale, and a quick temperature check confirmed a high fever. She was clammy to the touch, and her neck was stiff. Classic signs of meningitis were all there: the fever, the altered mental state, and the nuchal rigidity.

First things first, I had to secure her airway. I positioned her head correctly to ensure that her tongue wouldn't block her airway and checked for any obstructions. Her breathing, although shallow, was steady enough for now. I hooked her up to an oxygen mask to

make sure she was getting enough oxygen. I took out my flashlight and checked her pupils—both were reactive, which was a small relief.

Next, I needed to establish IV access. I grabbed a tourniquet and found a good vein in her arm. With practiced precision, I inserted the IV and started a saline drip. Hydration was crucial, especially with the fever she had. Fluids would help stabilize her a bit and make her more comfortable during the transport.

Her dorm mate hovered in the doorway, looking like she was about to faint. I gave her a quick glance and she blurted out that the patient had been complaining of a severe headache and neck pain for the past two days, but they had chalked it up to stress and poor posture from studying. It wasn't until she found her unconscious that she realized something was seriously wrong.

I needed to move fast. I did a quick full-body check for any other signs of injury or symptoms. No rashes that I could see, which was a bit unusual for bacterial meningitis, but not unheard of. Her blood pressure was low, heart rate was high—definitely signs of shock setting in. I relayed this information to my partner, who was preparing the stretcher outside.

We carefully transferred her to the stretcher, making sure to keep her head and neck stabilized. As we wheeled her out, the usual crowd had gathered, whis-

pering and taking videos. I ignored them. My focus was solely on the patient. We loaded her into the ambulance, and I hopped in beside her.

I started the sirens, and we took off. The patient's condition was critical, and every minute counted. I monitored her vitals closely. Blood pressure still low, heart rate still high, and her temperature wasn't budging. I administered a dose of broad-spectrum antibiotics through the IV. With suspected bacterial meningitis, you couldn't wait for a hospital diagnosis. Time was brain, quite literally.

As we sped through the streets, I kept a close eye on her. Her breathing started to become more labored, so I assisted with a bag-valve mask to ensure she was getting enough oxygen. I glanced at the clock—still at least ten minutes to the hospital. It felt like an eternity. I silently urged the ambulance to go faster.

I did another quick neuro check. Her pupils were still reactive, but she showed no response to pain stimuli. I checked her reflexes—none. Things were deteriorating fast. I had to be ready for anything. I prepped the equipment for intubation, just in case her breathing worsened.

To lighten the mood, if only for myself, I thought about how college students had this knack for waiting until the absolute worst moment to get seriously ill.

Midterms, finals, spring break—never a dull moment in campus life. I had seen it all, from drunken injuries to stress-induced fainting. But meningitis? That was a curveball.

The patient's condition wasn't improving, but it wasn't getting worse either. We were stabilizing, or at least holding steady. The hospital was in sight now. I radioed ahead to the ER, giving them a rundown of the patient's condition and our estimated arrival time. They were ready for us, thank goodness.

We pulled into the hospital bay, and the ER team was waiting with a gurney. We quickly transferred the patient over, giving the doctors a brief but detailed report on what we had done and observed. They rushed her inside, and I stepped back, my job done for now.

I took a deep breath and wiped the sweat off my forehead. It had been a tense ride, but we had made it. I felt a small sense of relief knowing that she was in good hands now. As I packed up the gear and prepped the ambulance for the next call, I couldn't help but think about the unpredictability of this job. One minute, you're dealing with a sprained ankle; the next, you're fighting to save a life.

As I hopped back into the ambulance, my partner gave me a knowing look. No words were needed. We both knew this was just another day in the life of a para-

medic. We headed back to the station, ready for whatever the next call would bring, knowing that we had done everything we could for the patient in the dorm room.

———

CRAZY AMBULANCE STORIES

CHAPTER TWELVE
HIT AND RUN

The paramedics brought in a man who had been run over by a truck and left for dead on the side of the road. He arrived unconscious and barely breathing, covered in dirt and blood. His clothes were torn, and the stark reality of his injuries was immediately apparent.

As the emergency room team rushed to stabilize him, I quickly assessed the situation. The patient had multiple lacerations, contusions, and suspected fractures. His left leg was mangled, and the lower half was twisted at an unnatural angle, indicating a severe compound fracture. His vital signs were unstable, with a blood pressure reading of 80/40 mmHg, a heart rate of 130 beats per minute, and shallow, rapid respirations at 30 breaths per minute. His Glasgow Coma Scale score

was 6, reflecting a severe head injury and a depressed level of consciousness.

First, we focused on airway management. The patient's airway was compromised due to facial trauma and potential cervical spine injury. We intubated him to secure the airway and provided mechanical ventilation. A cervical collar was applied to stabilize the neck and prevent any further spinal damage.

Next, we inserted two large-bore IV lines and began fluid resuscitation with normal saline to combat the hypovolemic shock caused by significant blood loss. We also administered blood products, starting with type O-negative blood until cross-matched blood became available. The patient required a massive transfusion protocol, given the extent of his injuries and ongoing blood loss.

While the nurses continued fluid resuscitation, I conducted a secondary survey to identify other life-threatening injuries. The patient's abdomen was distended and tender, raising concern for internal bleeding. A FAST (Focused Assessment with Sonography for Trauma) exam revealed free fluid in the abdomen, likely from a ruptured organ. We also noted decreased breath sounds on the right side, and a chest X-ray confirmed a hemothorax and multiple rib fractures.

We quickly inserted a chest tube on the right side to drain the accumulated blood and allow the lung to re-expand. The patient was also placed on a cardiac monitor, and we administered analgesics and sedatives to manage pain and agitation.

Due to the complexity of his injuries, we needed to prioritize the most critical interventions. The orthopedic surgeon was called in to evaluate the severely injured leg. After assessing the damage, it was clear that the patient would need emergent surgery to repair the compound fracture and attempt limb salvage. However, before any surgical intervention, he required stabilization in the operating room (OR).

The patient was prepped for emergency laparotomy to address the intra-abdominal bleeding. The general surgery team took over, and I remained in the OR to assist and monitor the patient's overall status. During the laparotomy, the surgeons discovered a ruptured spleen and multiple liver lacerations, which they swiftly repaired. They also controlled the hemorrhage and packed the abdomen temporarily to stabilize the patient.

With the abdominal bleeding controlled, the orthopedic team began their work on the leg. They performed an external fixation to stabilize the fractured bones and prevent further damage to the surrounding tissues.

Given the extent of the soft tissue injury, a definitive repair would be deferred until the patient was more stable and the risk of infection was minimized.

Post-operatively, the patient was transferred to the intensive care unit (ICU) for close monitoring and continued resuscitation. In the ICU, he remained on mechanical ventilation, and we continued aggressive fluid and blood product administration. We also initiated broad-spectrum antibiotics to prevent infection, given the open fractures and extensive soft tissue damage.

Throughout the next 48 hours, the patient's condition remained critical but gradually improved with meticulous care. We monitored his neurological status closely, given the initial low Glasgow Coma Scale score. A CT scan of the head revealed a subdural hematoma, which was evacuated by the neurosurgery team. His intracranial pressure was monitored with an intracranial pressure (ICP) monitor to ensure there was no further swelling or bleeding.

Pain management was a crucial aspect of his care, as the multiple fractures and surgical interventions caused significant discomfort. We used a combination of intravenous opioids and regional nerve blocks to control his pain while minimizing the risk of respiratory depression. Additionally, we implemented a strict physio-

therapy regimen to prevent complications such as deep vein thrombosis and pulmonary embolism, which are common in patients with severe trauma and prolonged immobility.

Infection control was another priority. The open fracture and surgical sites were meticulously cleaned and dressed regularly. We cultured the wounds to identify any potential pathogens and adjusted the antibiotic therapy based on culture results. The patient received a tetanus prophylaxis given the nature of his injuries.

The patient remained in the ICU for a week, during which his condition gradually stabilized. He was slowly weaned off the mechanical ventilator and transitioned to supplemental oxygen via nasal cannula. His renal function, initially compromised due to shock, improved with careful monitoring of fluid balance and renal protective strategies.

After a week in the ICU, the patient was stable enough to be transferred to a surgical step-down unit. Here, the focus shifted to rehabilitation and further surgical planning. The orthopedic team performed a definitive fixation of the leg fracture and addressed any remaining soft tissue injuries. This involved multiple surgeries, including debridement and skin grafts, to ensure proper healing and minimize the risk of infection.

Throughout his recovery, the patient required intensive physical and occupational therapy. The road to regaining full functionality was long and arduous, but with the support of a multidisciplinary team, significant progress was made. He learned to use assistive devices to aid mobility and participated in strength-building exercises to regain muscle mass and improve overall endurance.

Psychological support was also an integral part of his rehabilitation. The trauma of the accident, combined with the prolonged hospital stay and uncertainty about the future, took a toll on his mental health. Counseling and support from a dedicated psychiatric team helped him cope with the emotional challenges and fostered a positive outlook on his recovery.

The patient's journey through the emergency room and subsequent treatment was a testament to the resilience of the human body and the importance of a coordinated, multidisciplinary approach in trauma care. Despite the severity of his injuries and the initial prognosis, he defied the odds and embarked on a long but promising road to recovery.

After several months of intensive rehabilitation and numerous follow-up appointments, the patient was discharged home. He continued outpatient physical therapy and attended regular check-ups to monitor his

progress. The road to full recovery was still ahead, but the worst was behind him.

Reflecting on this case, I was reminded of the fragility of life and the incredible strength and determination that patients often exhibit in the face of adversity. The coordinated efforts of the emergency room team, surgeons, intensivists, nurses, and rehabilitation specialists played a crucial role in saving this patient's life and setting him on a path to recovery. It was a humbling and inspiring experience, one that reinforced my commitment to providing the best possible care to those in need.

CHAPTER THIRTEEN
SNAKE BITE

It was mid-July, the peak of summer, and the heat outside was relentless. I had just finished examining a patient with a severe case of heatstroke when I received a call from the paramedics. They were bringing in a patient who had been bitten by a rattlesnake.

The patient arrived swiftly, transported on a gurney with an oxygen mask covering his face. He was a middle-aged man, seemingly fit, but his distress was evident. The paramedics relayed that he had been bitten on the right forearm while gardening in his backyard. They had administered basic first aid, including immobilizing the affected limb and providing supplemental oxygen.

I quickly assessed the patient's condition. His skin was pale and clammy, and he was sweating profusely.

His breathing was rapid and shallow, and his pulse was thready, indicating that his cardiovascular system was under severe stress. The bite site on his forearm was swollen and showed the characteristic fang marks. The surrounding tissue was already showing signs of erythema and edema, extending up towards his elbow.

I ordered a series of immediate interventions and diagnostic tests. First, I had an IV line inserted to administer fluids to combat hypotension and prevent shock. I requested a complete blood count (CBC), coagulation profile, serum electrolytes, renal function tests, and a baseline electrocardiogram (ECG). Given the nature of the injury, I also ordered a dose of polyvalent crotaline Fab antivenom, which is effective against North American pit viper envenomations, to be prepared.

While waiting for the antivenom to arrive, I continued to monitor the patient's vitals closely. His blood pressure was dangerously low at 80/50 mmHg, and his heart rate was elevated at 120 beats per minute. I initiated a normal saline infusion to address the hypotension and ensure adequate perfusion of his organs. The initial blood tests revealed a marked leukocytosis, indicating a systemic inflammatory response, and a coagulopathy with an elevated prothrombin time (PT) and partial thromboplastin time (PTT), suggesting

that the venom had started to interfere with his blood's ability to clot.

The antivenom arrived within minutes, and I administered it intravenously, starting with an initial dose of four vials. Antivenom therapy is critical in neutralizing the venom and preventing further systemic damage. The infusion was closely monitored for any signs of an allergic reaction, which can occur despite pretreatment with antihistamines and corticosteroids. Fortunately, the patient tolerated the infusion well, and I continued to administer fluids to support his circulatory system.

As the antivenom began to take effect, I noticed a gradual improvement in the patient's condition. His blood pressure started to stabilize, and his heart rate began to decrease. However, the swelling in his arm continued to progress, now extending to his upper arm and shoulder. This indicated that the local effects of the venom were still active, necessitating further doses of antivenom.

I administered an additional two vials of antivenom and closely monitored the patient for signs of compartment syndrome, a serious complication where increased pressure within a muscle compartment can impede blood flow and cause tissue death. To ensure this condition did not develop, I measured the circum-

ference of his affected arm at regular intervals and monitored for any signs of increased pain, paresthesia, or pallor.

Over the next few hours, the patient's condition continued to stabilize. His blood pressure normalized, and his heart rate settled into a more manageable rhythm. The swelling in his arm began to subside, and the erythema and edema showed signs of improvement. However, the patient's coagulation profile remained abnormal, with persistent elevated PT and PTT levels, indicating that the venom's effects on his blood clotting were ongoing.

Given the severity of the envenomation and the patient's unstable coagulation status, I decided to transfer him to the intensive care unit (ICU) for continuous monitoring and further management. In the ICU, he would receive additional doses of antivenom as needed, along with supportive care to address any complications that might arise.

The treatment plan in the ICU included continued administration of antivenom until his coagulation parameters returned to normal and the swelling in his arm subsided completely. He was also given broad-spectrum antibiotics prophylactically to prevent secondary bacterial infection at the bite site, along with analgesics to manage his pain.

The patient's renal function was monitored closely due to the risk of acute kidney injury from the myotoxic effects of the venom and the large volumes of fluids administered. His urine output was measured hourly, and his serum creatinine levels were checked regularly.

By the second day in the ICU, the patient's coagulation profile began to show signs of improvement, and the swelling in his arm had significantly decreased. He remained hemodynamically stable, and his renal function tests were within normal limits. The patient was gradually weaned off the IV fluids as his condition improved, and his pain was well-controlled with oral analgesics.

On the third day, the patient was stable enough to be transferred out of the ICU to a regular medical ward. His coagulation profile had normalized, and the swelling in his arm had almost completely resolved. He continued to receive physical therapy to regain full function of his arm, which had been immobilized for several days.

By the end of the week, the patient was well enough to be discharged. He was given detailed instructions on wound care and a follow-up appointment with a hematologist to monitor his coagulation status. He was also prescribed a course of oral antibiotics to complete at

home and instructed to avoid any strenuous activity until he had fully recovered.

The patient returned for his follow-up appointment two weeks later, showing no signs of infection or complications. His coagulation profile remained normal, and he had regained full function of his arm. He expressed gratitude for the care he had received and was eager to return to his normal activities.

CHAPTER FOURTEEN
COVID

It was an ordinary shift in the emergency room, though 'ordinary' is a relative term in the chaos of the ER. As an emergency room doctor, I had grown accustomed to the unpredictable nature of the job. On this particular day, a middle-aged woman was wheeled in on a gurney, her body shaking with the effort to breathe. She was obese, her frame straining against the confines of the stretcher, and her labored breathing was a stark reminder of the severity of her condition.

The patient had severe COVID-19, a diagnosis that had become all too common over the past months. Her chart indicated that she had been symptomatic for over a week, with progressive shortness of breath, fever, and a persistent cough. Her oxygen saturation levels were

critically low at 82%, and she was visibly cyanotic, her lips and fingertips tinged with blue.

The first priority was stabilizing her breathing. We placed her on high-flow nasal cannula oxygen therapy, delivering 60 liters per minute with an FiO2 of 100%. Despite this, her oxygen saturation levels struggled to climb above 85%. Her respiratory rate was alarmingly high at 30 breaths per minute, and her chest heaved with each inhalation.

A thorough examination revealed bilateral coarse crackles on auscultation, indicative of widespread lung involvement. Her heart rate was tachycardic at 120 beats per minute, and her blood pressure was elevated at 160/95 mmHg. Given her obesity, her body mass index (BMI) was calculated to be 42, placing her in the morbidly obese category. This added a significant layer of complexity to her management, as obesity is a known risk factor for severe COVID-19 outcomes.

A rapid assessment was conducted, and blood tests were ordered, including a complete blood count (CBC), metabolic panel, coagulation profile, D-dimer, and inflammatory markers such as C-reactive protein (CRP) and ferritin. A chest X-ray was also ordered, which revealed bilateral diffuse infiltrates consistent with COVID-19 pneumonia. Given the severity of her symp-

toms, we proceeded with a computed tomography (CT) scan of the chest, which confirmed extensive ground-glass opacities and consolidation.

The patient's condition warranted aggressive intervention. We initiated intravenous corticosteroids, administering dexamethasone 6 mg daily, which has been shown to reduce mortality in severe COVID-19 cases. Additionally, given her elevated D-dimer levels, indicative of a hypercoagulable state, we started her on prophylactic anticoagulation with enoxaparin 40 mg subcutaneously daily to prevent thromboembolic events.

Fluid management was crucial, especially considering her obesity and the risk of fluid overload. We maintained a conservative fluid strategy, carefully balancing hydration to avoid worsening her pulmonary edema. Intravenous fluids were administered judiciously, and her urine output was closely monitored.

Given the high likelihood of bacterial superinfection in severe cases, broad-spectrum antibiotics were initiated empirically. Ceftriaxone 1 gram daily and azithromycin 500 mg daily were chosen based on her clinical presentation and local antibiogram data. Blood and sputum cultures were also obtained to tailor antibiotic therapy based on culture results.

As her respiratory status remained precarious, we consulted the intensive care unit (ICU) team early in her management. The decision was made to escalate her respiratory support. She was transitioned to non-invasive positive pressure ventilation (NIPPV) with bilevel positive airway pressure (BiPAP). The initial settings were an inspiratory positive airway pressure (IPAP) of 15 cm H2O and an expiratory positive airway pressure (EPAP) of 10 cm H2O, with 100% oxygen.

Despite these efforts, her condition continued to deteriorate. Her arterial blood gases (ABG) showed worsening hypoxemia and hypercapnia, with a PaO2 of 55 mmHg and a PaCO2 of 60 mmHg. The ICU team was called in, and after discussing the case, it was clear that intubation and mechanical ventilation were necessary to prevent impending respiratory failure.

The intubation was challenging due to her obesity, requiring careful planning and the use of a video laryngoscope for better visualization of her airway. Once intubated, she was placed on a mechanical ventilator with a lung-protective strategy: a tidal volume of 6 ml/kg of predicted body weight, a positive end-expiratory pressure (PEEP) of 10 cm H2O, and an FiO2 titrated to maintain oxygen saturation above 90%.

Given her critical condition, we initiated a contin-

uous infusion of vasopressors to support her blood pressure. Norepinephrine was started at 0.05 mcg/kg/min and titrated based on her hemodynamic response. Sedation was maintained with propofol and fentanyl to ensure comfort and compliance with the ventilator.

In parallel, we addressed her metabolic needs. A nasogastric tube was placed for enteral feeding, and a detailed nutrition plan was developed with the assistance of a dietitian, considering her obesity and the need for adequate caloric and protein intake to support her recovery.

Laboratory results indicated elevated inflammatory markers, with a CRP of 200 mg/L and ferritin of 1500 ng/mL, signifying a severe inflammatory response. To address this, we considered immunomodulatory therapy. Tocilizumab, an interleukin-6 receptor antagonist, was administered at a dose of 8 mg/kg, given the emerging evidence of its benefit in severe COVID-19 cases with hyperinflammation.

Throughout her time in the ER, the patient's condition was closely monitored. Regular ABGs, chest X-rays, and laboratory tests were conducted to assess her response to treatment and adjust the management plan accordingly. Despite these intensive efforts, her prog-

nosis remained guarded due to the severity of her illness and underlying comorbidities.

After several hours of stabilization and aggressive management in the ER, the patient was transferred to the ICU for ongoing care. The transition was smooth, and the ICU team was well-briefed on her condition and the interventions that had been initiated.

In the ICU, her condition continued to be critical but stable. The multidisciplinary team, including pulmonologists, intensivists, and infectious disease specialists, worked collaboratively to optimize her care. Over the next several days, her progress was slow, with small signs of improvement. Her oxygenation gradually stabilized, and inflammatory markers began to trend downwards.

However, her journey was far from over. The risk of complications remained high, and she required prolonged mechanical ventilation and supportive care. The team remained vigilant for secondary infections, renal dysfunction, and other potential issues that could arise during her prolonged ICU stay.

Ultimately, the patient's story in the ER was a testament to the complexity and severity of severe COVID-19 in patients with significant comorbidities. The multifaceted approach, including respiratory support, pharmacological intervention, and meticulous monitor-

ing, highlighted the critical role of the emergency room in the initial management of such life-threatening cases. Whether she would ultimately survive the ordeal was uncertain, but the comprehensive and aggressive management in the ER had given her the best possible chance.

CHAPTER FIFTEEN
SEVERE BURNS

It was a hectic Monday evening in the emergency room, the kind of night where the beds filled faster than we could discharge patients. I had just completed a particularly exhausting shift when the triage nurse approached me with urgency in her eyes. She handed me the chart for a teenage boy who had just arrived with severe burns on his left arm from a boiling pot of water. The initial report suggested extensive damage, and I knew this case would demand immediate and thorough attention.

I approached the patient, who lay on the gurney with his left arm cradled protectively against his chest. The boy was visibly in shock, his face pale and contorted with pain. The burn covered a significant

portion of his forearm, extending from just below the elbow to the wrist. The skin was a ghastly mix of bright red and blistering white, indicating a combination of second and third-degree burns.

I began with a rapid assessment to determine the extent of the burns and to check for any other injuries. The skin on his arm was swollen and blistered, with patches where the epidermis had sloughed off, revealing the underlying dermis. In some areas, the burn had penetrated deeper, reaching the subcutaneous tissues. I carefully palpated the arm, noting the absence of hair and the leathery texture indicative of full-thickness burns. The severity of the injury required immediate intervention to prevent further damage and complications.

The first step in the treatment plan was to alleviate the patient's pain and stabilize his condition. I administered intravenous morphine to manage his pain, which was crucial for both his comfort and our ability to proceed with further treatment. Next, I set up an IV line to ensure he remained hydrated and to facilitate the administration of medications. Given the extent of the burns, I ordered a tetanus booster to prevent infection, as the damaged skin provided a potential entry point for bacteria.

With the initial pain management underway, I proceeded to clean the burn area. Using sterile saline, I gently irrigated the wound to remove any debris and residual boiling water. The patient's discomfort was palpable, but the morphine had begun to take effect, dulling the edge of his pain. After cleaning the wound, I applied a topical antibiotic ointment to prevent infection and covered the burn with a sterile, non-adherent dressing to protect the area from further trauma and contamination.

To monitor for signs of systemic infection or other complications, I ordered a series of blood tests, including a complete blood count (CBC) and a metabolic panel. The results would provide insight into the patient's overall condition and help us anticipate potential issues that might arise during his treatment. I also requested a set of X-rays to rule out any underlying fractures or other injuries that might have occurred during the accident.

As the team worked to stabilize the patient, I began to consider the long-term management of his burns. The extent and depth of the injuries would likely require specialized care that we could not provide in the emergency room. I contacted the burn unit at a nearby hospital with a dedicated team of burn specialists. They

had the facilities and expertise to handle severe cases like this one, offering a better chance for optimal recovery.

After coordinating with the burn unit, we prepared the patient for transfer. In the meantime, I continued to monitor his vital signs, ensuring that his pain was controlled and that there were no signs of respiratory distress or circulatory compromise. Burns of this severity can lead to significant fluid loss and electrolyte imbalances, so it was crucial to keep a close watch on his condition.

Once the transfer was confirmed, I briefed the transport team on the patient's condition, the treatments administered, and the plan for ongoing care. I also made sure to include detailed notes on his chart for the receiving team, outlining the severity of the burns, the areas affected, and the treatments provided thus far.

The patient was transported to the burn unit without incident, and I followed up with the receiving team to ensure a smooth transition of care. They reported that the boy was stable upon arrival and that they would begin a comprehensive treatment plan that included surgical debridement, skin grafts, and ongoing wound care. The specialized care at the burn unit would significantly increase his chances of a successful recov-

ery, although the road ahead would be long and challenging.

Over the next few days, I checked in with the burn unit to track the patient's progress. The team informed me that he had undergone his first debridement surgery, which involved the removal of dead and damaged tissue to promote healing and prevent infection. The procedure had gone well, and they were optimistic about his recovery, although they cautioned that it would take time and multiple surgeries to fully address the extent of his injuries.

The patient's treatment plan included daily wound care, pain management, and physical therapy to maintain mobility and prevent contractures, which are a common complication of severe burns. The burn unit's multidisciplinary approach, involving surgeons, nurses, physical therapists, and psychologists, ensured that all aspects of his recovery were addressed, from the physical healing of his burns to the emotional and psychological impact of his injury.

As the days turned into weeks, the patient continued to make progress. He underwent several more surgeries to graft healthy skin onto the burned areas, a painstaking process that required meticulous care to ensure the grafts took hold and began to integrate with his existing tissue. The physical therapy

sessions, though painful and exhausting, were crucial in maintaining the range of motion in his arm and preventing the formation of scar tissue that could limit his mobility.

The burn unit kept me updated on his progress, and I was heartened to hear that the patient was responding well to treatment. The risk of infection, a significant concern with burns of this severity, was being managed effectively with the use of antibiotics and rigorous wound care protocols. His pain was also being managed with a combination of medications and therapies designed to minimize discomfort while avoiding the pitfalls of long-term opioid use.

Months later, I received a final update from the burn unit. The patient had been discharged and was continuing his recovery at home with regular outpatient visits to the burn clinic. He had regained a significant amount of function in his arm, although he would require ongoing physical therapy and follow-up surgeries to address the scarring and improve his range of motion further. The emotional impact of his injury was also being addressed through counseling, helping him to cope with the trauma and the long journey of recovery ahead.

Each step, from pain management and wound care to the coordination of his transfer and the follow-up

treatments, played a crucial role in his journey toward healing.

As an emergency room doctor, it was a privilege to be a part of this young boy's recovery, witnessing first-hand the impact of dedicated and compassionate care in the face of such a devastating injury.

CHAPTER SIXTEEN
SYSTEMIC INFECTION

The shift had been fairly routine until a middle-aged woman was wheeled into the emergency room on a gurney. According to the paramedics, she had fainted multiple times at home. She was conscious but appeared lethargic and confused. The initial assessment began with taking her vital signs. Her blood pressure was alarmingly low, her heart rate was elevated, and her temperature was slightly above normal. She seemed pale and clammy, which was concerning. Fainting episodes can be caused by a variety of factors, but her symptoms suggested a potentially serious underlying condition.

I ordered an immediate ECG to check for any cardiac irregularities. The results showed sinus tachycardia, which was expected given her elevated heart rate but

did not provide a clear cause for her fainting spells. Given her symptoms, I considered a broad differential diagnosis that included cardiac, neurological, and metabolic causes.

The next step was a thorough physical examination. Her abdomen was tender, particularly in the lower quadrants, and she winced when I palpated near her lower right rib cage. Her skin showed no signs of trauma or bruising, but I noted a small, red, swollen area on her thigh, which appeared to be a possible site of infection. I decided to draw blood for a complete blood count (CBC), blood cultures, and a metabolic panel, and to perform a urinalysis to rule out any infections or metabolic imbalances.

While waiting for the laboratory results, I administered intravenous fluids to address her low blood pressure and tachycardia. Given her presentation and the lack of an immediate clear cause, I also started broad-spectrum antibiotics, specifically vancomycin and piperacillin-tazobactam, to cover a wide range of possible bacterial infections. This was a precautionary measure to combat any potential sepsis, which was a serious concern given her low blood pressure and elevated heart rate.

The lab results came back within the hour. Her white blood cell count was significantly elevated, indi-

cating an infection. Blood cultures were not yet available, but her urinalysis showed no signs of a urinary tract infection. Her metabolic panel was unremarkable except for a slightly elevated creatinine level, suggesting possible dehydration or early kidney dysfunction. The CBC also showed a marked increase in inflammatory markers, which reinforced the suspicion of a systemic infection.

Given the physical findings and lab results, I ordered imaging studies to further investigate the source of her infection. A chest X-ray showed no signs of pneumonia, but a CT scan of her abdomen and pelvis revealed inflammation and fluid collection around her liver, consistent with an abscess. This finding correlated with the tenderness she exhibited during the physical examination and explained her systemic symptoms.

I consulted with the surgery and infectious disease teams. The consensus was that she likely had a staph infection that had disseminated, leading to the liver abscess and her systemic symptoms. The small, red, swollen area on her thigh was suspected to be the primary site of the staph infection, possibly from a minor injury or unnoticed cut that had become infected.

The patient was transferred to the intensive care unit (ICU) for closer monitoring and aggressive treatment. The treatment plan included continued adminis-

tration of broad-spectrum antibiotics, with a switch to more targeted antibiotics once the blood culture results identified the specific strain of Staphylococcus. We initiated a regimen of intravenous vancomycin for MRSA coverage and adjusted the dose based on her kidney function. She was also given intravenous fluids to maintain her blood pressure and support her renal function.

Given the presence of a liver abscess, surgical intervention was necessary. The surgery team performed a percutaneous drainage of the abscess under ultrasound guidance. This procedure involved inserting a needle through her skin into the abscess to drain the infected fluid. The drained fluid was sent for culture and sensitivity testing to guide further antibiotic therapy.

Post-procedure, the patient remained in the ICU for close monitoring. Her blood pressure gradually stabilized with fluid resuscitation and vasopressors, and her heart rate normalized. The results from the abscess fluid culture confirmed the presence of Staphylococcus aureus, and fortunately, it was sensitive to vancomycin, affirming our choice of antibiotics.

Over the next few days, her condition improved steadily. The inflammatory markers in her blood tests began to decrease, indicating that the infection was responding to the antibiotics. Her fever resolved, and she became more alert and oriented. The drainage

catheter remained in place to allow continuous drainage of the abscess, reducing the risk of recurrent infection.

Throughout her ICU stay, we continued to monitor her kidney function, adjusting her fluid and electrolyte balance as necessary. She required physical therapy to regain strength due to prolonged bed rest and the systemic effects of the infection. The infection control team emphasized strict hygiene measures to prevent any further hospital-acquired infections.

After about a week in the ICU, her condition had stabilized sufficiently for transfer to a regular medical ward. She continued to receive intravenous antibiotics and underwent regular blood tests to monitor her progress. The catheter for abscess drainage was removed once imaging confirmed that the abscess had resolved.

The patient was eventually discharged from the hospital with a prescription for oral antibiotics to complete a full course of treatment, and follow-up appointments were scheduled with the infectious disease and surgery teams. Instructions were provided for wound care and signs of potential complications, emphasizing the importance of completing the antibiotic course to prevent recurrence of the infection.

In follow-up visits, the patient showed no signs of

recurrent infection. Her liver function tests normalized, and there were no residual signs of abscess on follow-up imaging. The infection site on her thigh healed without complications, though she was advised to watch for any new symptoms and to maintain good hygiene to prevent future infections.

The patient's recovery was a testament to the importance of prompt and aggressive treatment of systemic infections. Her initial presentation with fainting and systemic symptoms could have led to a multitude of diagnoses, but a thorough and methodical approach to her assessment, diagnosis, and treatment ensured a positive outcome. Despite the severity of her condition, she made a full recovery thanks to the collaborative efforts of the emergency, surgical, and infectious disease teams.

CHAPTER SEVENTEEN
SPIDER BITE

It was a typically hectic night in the emergency room, a relentless barrage of injuries, illnesses, and crises. The dim, artificial light cast a sterile glow over the bustling space, a backdrop for the symphony of beeping monitors and the soft murmur of concerned voices. My shift had barely begun when the call came in: a patient en route, possible black widow spider bite. As an emergency room doctor, I'd seen my share of venomous bites, but black widows always commanded a certain level of respect. Their venom was potent, their bite often debilitating.

The patient arrived via ambulance, a middle-aged individual, their face contorted in pain. Paramedics briefed me quickly: the bite had occurred approximately three hours earlier while the patient was cleaning out

their garage. Initial symptoms were mild, but within the last hour, they had escalated significantly.

I began my assessment, noting the patient's symptoms: severe muscle cramping, particularly in the abdomen, which they described as the worst pain they'd ever experienced. Their blood pressure was elevated, heart rate rapid, and they were sweating profusely despite the air-conditioned room. The patient also reported nausea and dizziness, all classic signs of envenomation by Latrodectus mactans, the black widow spider.

The bite site itself was on the lower leg, a small, red puncture mark surrounded by a halo of erythema. There was some swelling, but nothing that immediately suggested necrosis or severe local reaction. Black widow venom works systemically, disrupting nerve function and causing widespread symptoms rather than local tissue damage.

I ordered a series of tests to rule out other possible causes for the symptoms and to assess the patient's overall condition. Blood work would check for signs of infection or other systemic issues, while an ECG would monitor cardiac function, given the elevated heart rate and blood pressure. A comprehensive metabolic panel would help determine if the venom was affecting the kidneys or liver.

While waiting for the test results, I moved quickly to manage the patient's symptoms and prevent complications. Pain management was a priority. I administered intravenous opioids, titrating the dose carefully to relieve the patient's intense pain without causing excessive sedation or respiratory depression. Muscle relaxants, such as diazepam, were also given to help alleviate the severe cramping.

To address the elevated blood pressure and heart rate, I prescribed a beta-blocker, such as metoprolol. This would help to stabilize the cardiovascular system and reduce the risk of arrhythmias. Antiemetics were administered to combat the nausea, and I ensured the patient was well-hydrated with intravenous fluids, which would also support their cardiovascular system and help flush the venom from their body.

As the medications began to take effect, the patient's pain gradually diminished, and their heart rate and blood pressure started to stabilize. The blood tests came back largely normal, aside from slightly elevated white blood cell counts, likely a stress response to the severe pain and venom. The ECG showed no immediate signs of cardiac distress, which was a good sign.

Despite the improvement, I remained vigilant. Black widow envenomation can cause a condition known as latrodectism, which can lead to complications such as

rhabdomyolysis (breakdown of muscle tissue) or renal failure in severe cases. Monitoring the patient's kidney function was crucial. I ordered urine tests to check for myoglobin, a marker of muscle breakdown, and continued to monitor their vital signs closely.

As the hours passed, the patient's condition continued to improve. The pain was now manageable with oral medications, and the muscle cramps had subsided significantly. Their vital signs were stable, and there were no signs of complications from the venom.

The next step was to address the bite itself. Although the systemic symptoms were the primary concern, it was essential to ensure that the bite site did not become infected. I cleaned the wound thoroughly and applied a topical antibiotic ointment. Given the patient's overall good health and lack of complicating factors like diabetes or immunosuppression, I decided against prescribing systemic antibiotics, instead opting for close monitoring and good wound care.

The patient was admitted for overnight observation. This allowed for continued pain management and monitoring for any delayed complications. By the next morning, the patient was much improved. Their pain was minimal, their vital signs stable, and there were no signs of renal or cardiac complications.

Before discharge, I provided detailed instructions

for home care. The patient was to continue taking pain medications as needed, but to switch to over-the-counter options like ibuprofen or acetaminophen if the pain remained mild. I also advised them to take a muscle relaxant if they experienced any residual cramping. I stressed the importance of staying hydrated and monitoring their urine output for any signs of kidney issues, such as dark or reduced urine.

Additionally, the patient was instructed to keep the bite site clean and dry, applying antibiotic ointment daily and covering it with a sterile bandage. They were to watch for signs of infection, such as increased redness, swelling, or discharge, and to seek medical attention if these occurred.

I scheduled a follow-up appointment for the patient in two days to reassess their condition and ensure there were no delayed complications. Before they left, I took a moment to emphasize the importance of avoiding future encounters with spiders, particularly in cluttered or storage areas like their garage. Simple precautions, such as wearing gloves and long sleeves, could significantly reduce the risk of another bite.

Over the next few days, I checked in on the patient via phone calls. They reported steady improvement, with only occasional mild cramping and no new symptoms. When they returned for their follow-up appoint-

ment, they were almost back to their normal self. The bite site was healing well, with no signs of infection, and their urine output remained normal, indicating healthy kidney function.

In the end, the patient made a full recovery. The prompt and appropriate treatment in the emergency room, combined with diligent follow-up care, had mitigated the potentially severe effects of the black widow spider venom.

CHAPTER EIGHTEEN
ALLERGIC REACTION

It was an unremarkable Thursday evening in the emergency room, the kind where the hum of fluorescent lights and the occasional murmur of staff punctuate the otherwise quiet night. I had just finished charting on my last patient when the call came in. A severe allergic reaction. The nurse's tone conveyed the urgency, and I immediately prepared myself for what was to come.

The patient arrived by ambulance, accompanied by frantic paramedics who quickly transferred him to the gurney in the triage area. As they wheeled him in, I could see the severity of his condition. His face was swollen, his lips were puffed and blue, and a red, blotchy rash spread across his neck and arms. He was gasping for breath, each inhale a desperate struggle. His airway was clearly compromised.

The paramedics handed me the brief history: the patient had accidentally ingested peanuts, despite knowing his severe allergy. He had quickly developed symptoms, and by the time the paramedics arrived, he was in full-blown anaphylaxis.

I directed the team to move the patient to a resuscitation bay. Time was critical. Anaphylaxis can escalate rapidly, leading to respiratory failure, shock, and death if not managed promptly. As we moved, I called out orders to the nurses. We needed epinephrine immediately, the cornerstone of anaphylactic treatment. I instructed the nurse to administer 0.3 mg of intramuscular epinephrine into the patient's thigh, the fastest route to get the drug into his system.

While the nurse administered the epinephrine, I assessed the patient's vitals. His blood pressure was dangerously low, 70/40 mmHg, indicating shock. His oxygen saturation was plummeting, reading 82% on room air. He was tachycardic, with a heart rate of 140 beats per minute, his body's response to the profound hypotension and hypoxia.

I ordered a high-flow oxygen mask to deliver 100% oxygen, hoping to improve his saturations. Simultaneously, I instructed another nurse to establish two large-bore intravenous lines. We needed access for fluids and medications. The nurse hung a liter of

normal saline and started it wide open to combat the hypotension.

The patient's tongue was swelling, further threatening his airway. I needed to secure his airway before it became completely obstructed. I called for the intubation kit and prepared for rapid sequence intubation (RSI). We administered etomidate for sedation and succinylcholine to paralyze his muscles, allowing for a smoother intubation process. With the patient sedated and paralyzed, I carefully inserted the endotracheal tube, guiding it past the swollen tissues and into the trachea. Once the tube was in place, I confirmed placement with auscultation and end-tidal CO_2 monitoring. His oxygen saturation improved to 94% once we started mechanical ventilation.

With the airway secure, I turned my attention to the ongoing anaphylactic reaction. Epinephrine was essential, but other medications were needed to stabilize the patient. I ordered an intravenous bolus of diphenhydramine, 50 mg, to counteract the histamine release. I also ordered 125 mg of methylprednisolone IV to reduce inflammation and prevent biphasic anaphylaxis, where symptoms can recur hours after the initial reaction. Additionally, I administered 50 mg of ranitidine IV to block H2 histamine receptors, complementing the H1 blockade provided by diphenhydramine.

Despite the initial interventions, the patient's blood pressure remained low. I ordered a continuous infusion of norepinephrine, starting at 0.1 mcg/kg/min, to maintain perfusion to vital organs. The nurse titrated the infusion to keep his mean arterial pressure above 65 mmHg.

As the patient's condition stabilized, I reviewed his history and medications. He had no other known medical conditions and was not taking any regular medications. His allergy to peanuts was well-documented, and he usually carried an epinephrine auto-injector, which he had used prior to the arrival of the paramedics. Despite his best efforts, the severity of his reaction overwhelmed the initial dose.

Over the next hour, the patient's condition began to improve. His blood pressure stabilized, and his oxygen saturation remained steady. The swelling in his face and airway started to subside, though it would take time for the edema to resolve completely. We continued to monitor him closely in the resuscitation bay, ready to intervene if he deteriorated.

Once he was stable, I arranged for him to be transferred to the intensive care unit (ICU) for ongoing monitoring. Anaphylaxis can have delayed or biphasic reactions, and I wanted to ensure he was in a setting where immediate care was available if needed. I

updated the ICU team on his status and the treatments administered.

In the ICU, the patient continued to receive supportive care. The norepinephrine infusion was gradually weaned as his blood pressure normalized. The steroids, antihistamines, and H2 blockers were continued to ensure complete resolution of the anaphylactic reaction. By the following morning, his condition had significantly improved. He was weaned off the ventilator and extubated successfully. His airway swelling had reduced enough to allow him to breathe comfortably on his own.

The ICU team monitored him for another 24 hours. During this time, he remained stable with no recurrence of symptoms. The steroids and antihistamines were tapered as his condition allowed. By the end of his ICU stay, he was transferred to a regular medical floor for observation and education on managing his severe allergy.

Before discharge, I met with the patient to discuss his condition and the steps he needed to take to prevent future episodes. We reviewed the importance of avoiding all peanut-containing products and the need to carry multiple epinephrine auto-injectors. I also referred him to an allergist for further evaluation and long-term management. The patient was profoundly

grateful for the care he received and determined to adhere strictly to his allergy management plan.

As an emergency physician, I am often the first line of defense in life-threatening situations. The patient's recovery was a testament to the power of modern medicine and the dedication of healthcare professionals.

CHAPTER NINETEEN
CHEMICAL EXPOSURE

The shift had started like any other, with the familiar bustle of the emergency room, patients coming in with various ailments and injuries. It wasn't long before the paramedics brought in a patient who would make this day unforgettable. The patient arrived on a stretcher, eyes half-closed, breathing labored. The paramedics relayed that the patient had been exposed to chemicals at a nearby plant, and the situation was critical.

Immediately, I noticed the telltale signs of chemical exposure. The patient's skin was flushed, and there were areas of blistering, particularly around the face and hands. The eyes were red and swollen, with clear signs of irritation. The patient was gasping for breath, indicating potential damage to the respiratory system.

As I took in these symptoms, the urgency of the situation became clear.

We moved the patient to a treatment room and initiated a rapid assessment. Vital signs were unstable: blood pressure was dangerously low, heart rate was elevated, and oxygen saturation levels were plummeting. The patient was also disoriented, likely due to hypoxia or possible neurotoxic effects of the chemical exposure.

The first step was to stabilize the patient. We administered high-flow oxygen via a non-rebreather mask to address the hypoxia. An IV line was quickly established, and fluids were administered to combat the hypotension. Given the possibility of a chemical burn, the patient was also given intravenous analgesics for pain management.

Next, we needed to identify the specific chemicals involved. The paramedics provided a crucial clue: the incident had occurred at a plant known for using chlorine and ammonia. Both chemicals could cause severe respiratory and skin damage, and the treatment protocols differed slightly. We decided to proceed with a broad-spectrum approach while awaiting confirmation.

A decontamination procedure was initiated to prevent further chemical absorption and protect the medical staff.

The patient's clothing was carefully removed, and the skin was thoroughly irrigated with copious amounts of water. This process was painstakingly slow, but it was necessary to mitigate the chemical's effects.

Once decontamination was complete, we turned our focus to more specific treatments. The patient's respiratory distress indicated a need for bronchodilators. We administered albuterol via a nebulizer to help open the airways. Additionally, corticosteroids were given to reduce inflammation in the lungs.

The patient's eye irritation was also a concern. We flushed the eyes with saline solution to remove any residual chemicals and prevent further damage. Ophthalmic antibiotics were administered prophylactically to prevent secondary infections.

As we continued treatment, the patient's condition remained critical. Blood tests and a chest X-ray were ordered to assess internal damage. The blood tests revealed elevated white blood cell counts, indicating a systemic inflammatory response. The chest X-ray showed pulmonary edema, a common complication of chemical inhalation.

To address the pulmonary edema, we administered diuretics to reduce fluid buildup in the lungs. Additionally, we started the patient on a broad-spectrum antibi-

otic regimen to prevent secondary infections, a common risk in cases of chemical exposure.

The patient's cardiovascular instability was another major concern. We administered vasopressors to maintain blood pressure and ensure adequate perfusion to vital organs. Continuous cardiac monitoring was essential to detect any arrhythmias that could arise from electrolyte imbalances.

Throughout the night, the patient's condition was touch and go. The critical care team was involved, and we worked tirelessly to stabilize the patient. Despite our best efforts, the patient's respiratory distress worsened. We made the decision to intubate and place the patient on mechanical ventilation to ensure adequate oxygenation.

In the following days, the patient's condition slowly began to improve. The inflammation in the lungs reduced, and the pulmonary edema started to resolve. The patient's blood pressure stabilized, and we were able to wean off the vasopressors. The skin lesions began to heal with the help of topical antibiotics and regular wound care.

However, the patient was not out of danger yet. The chemical exposure had caused significant damage to the liver and kidneys, likely due to the systemic inflammatory response. We monitored liver function tests and

renal function closely, adjusting medications as needed to support these organs.

The patient also required extensive physical therapy to recover from the muscle weakness and deconditioning caused by the prolonged critical illness. Nutritional support was provided via a feeding tube to ensure adequate caloric intake and promote healing.

Over the course of several weeks, the patient made remarkable progress. The mechanical ventilation was gradually reduced, and the patient was eventually extubated. Breathing remained labored, but it was significantly better than when the patient had first arrived. Pulmonary function tests indicated that while there was some permanent damage, the patient had regained a significant portion of lung capacity.

The psychological impact of the chemical exposure was also significant. The patient exhibited signs of posttraumatic stress disorder (PTSD), likely due to the traumatic experience and prolonged hospitalization. A referral to a mental health professional was made, and a treatment plan including counseling and medications was initiated to address these symptoms.

As the patient's condition continued to improve, we transitioned to an outpatient care plan. The patient was prescribed inhaled corticosteroids and bronchodilators to manage chronic lung inflammation. Oral antibiotics

were continued to prevent infections. Regular follow-ups with pulmonology and dermatology were scheduled to monitor the patient's progress and manage any long-term complications.

Reflecting on the case, it was clear that early intervention and aggressive treatment had been crucial in saving the patient's life. The collaboration among the emergency room team, critical care specialists, and various consultants had ensured a comprehensive approach to the patient's complex needs.

In the end, the patient was discharged with a good prognosis. There would be challenges ahead, with potential long-term effects on lung function and the psychological impact of the ordeal. However, the patient left the hospital with a renewed lease on life, a testament to the resilience of the human body and the dedication of the medical team.

This case underscored the importance of preparedness and swift action in managing chemical exposures. The lessons learned would undoubtedly enhance our ability to handle similar cases in the future, ensuring that we could provide the best possible care for those affected by such devastating events.

CHAPTER TWENTY
DVT

As I walked into the emergency room, the fluorescent lights buzzed quietly overhead, casting a sterile glow on the sea of bustling activity. Nurses hurried between patients, monitoring vital signs, administering medications, and charting progress. The scent of antiseptic was thick in the air, a constant reminder of the ongoing battle against infection and decay. I scanned the rows of beds, each occupied by individuals in various states of distress, and my eyes settled on a particularly concerning sight—a middle-aged man with a leg so swollen it seemed almost grotesque.

The patient was seated on the edge of a gurney, his face contorted in pain. His left leg was twice the size of his right, the skin stretched taut and a deep, angry red. From the knee down, the discoloration darkened to a

sinister purple, indicating the gravity of the situation. He had been brought in by a concerned neighbor, who mentioned that he had been complaining of leg pain for weeks but had stubbornly refused to seek medical help. Now, it was apparent that this delay could cost him dearly.

I approached the patient, noting the signs of distress etched into his features. The swollen leg was warm to the touch, almost feverish. A faint odor of necrosis began to emanate from the limb, suggesting that parts of the tissue were already dying. I palpated the leg gently, eliciting a sharp intake of breath from the patient. His calf was rock hard, a classic sign of a deep vein thrombosis (DVT) that had likely progressed to a severe state.

My initial diagnosis was that the patient was suffering from an advanced DVT, with potential complications of venous gangrene. This condition occurs when the blood clot in the deep veins obstructs blood flow so completely that the affected tissue starts to die from lack of oxygen and nutrients. The urgency of the situation was not lost on me; if left untreated, the clot could dislodge and travel to the lungs, causing a life-threatening pulmonary embolism.

To confirm my suspicions, I ordered an urgent Doppler ultrasound of the leg. This imaging test would

allow us to visualize the blood flow in the veins and identify the exact location and extent of the clot. While waiting for the radiology team, I started the patient on intravenous heparin, a fast-acting anticoagulant to prevent further clotting. I also ordered a complete blood count, coagulation profile, and renal function tests to assess the patient's overall health and readiness for more aggressive treatments.

The ultrasound results were as dire as I had anticipated. The clot extended from the mid-thigh down to the calf, completely occluding the venous return from the lower leg. The radiologist confirmed signs of tissue ischemia and early stages of necrosis, particularly in the foot and lower calf. The patient's prognosis was poor, and immediate intervention was required to salvage as much of the limb as possible and prevent systemic complications.

Given the severity of the clot and the extent of tissue damage, I discussed the case with the vascular surgery team. The consensus was to perform a thrombectomy, a surgical procedure to remove the clot and restore blood flow. In addition, we planned to administer thrombolytic therapy—powerful clot-dissolving drugs directly into the affected vein. This dual approach aimed to relieve the venous pressure and reduce the risk of further tissue death.

As we prepared the patient for surgery, I ensured he was well-hydrated and started him on broad-spectrum antibiotics to preempt any potential infections from the necrotic tissue. We also monitored his cardiovascular status closely, as patients with such extensive DVTs are at high risk for sudden cardiac events.

The surgical procedure was challenging. The vascular surgeon made an incision in the patient's thigh and carefully navigated to the site of the clot. Using specialized instruments, he extracted the thrombus piece by piece. Once the bulk of the clot was removed, a catheter was threaded into the vein to deliver the thrombolytic agents directly to the residual clot material. The entire process took several hours, during which we maintained a constant vigil on the patient's vital signs.

Post-operatively, the patient was transferred to the intensive care unit for close monitoring. We continued the anticoagulation therapy with heparin, transitioning to oral warfarin as his condition stabilized. Warfarin would help prevent new clots from forming while allowing us to monitor his blood's clotting ability regularly.

In addition to anticoagulation, we implemented a comprehensive wound care plan for the areas of necrosis. This included debridement of dead tissue, applica-

tion of topical antimicrobial agents, and frequent dressing changes. The goal was to promote healing and prevent infection, a constant threat in such cases.

The patient's recovery was slow and fraught with complications. The necrotic areas required repeated debridement, and there were times when it seemed the infection might overwhelm his immune system. We adjusted his antibiotic regimen based on culture results from the wound, ensuring we targeted any resistant bacteria effectively.

Physical therapy was also a critical component of his rehabilitation. The prolonged immobility and tissue damage had left his leg weak and stiff. Our physiotherapists worked with him daily, guiding him through exercises designed to restore strength and flexibility. This process was painful and frustrating for the patient, but he persevered, understanding that mobility was crucial to his overall recovery.

Throughout this ordeal, I couldn't help but reflect on the importance of timely medical intervention. The patient's stubbornness and delay in seeking help had nearly cost him his life and his limb. It was a stark reminder of the dangers of ignoring symptoms and the critical role of early detection and treatment in preventing severe outcomes.

Over the following weeks, the patient's condition

gradually improved. The swelling in his leg subsided, and the color began to return to a more natural hue. The areas of necrosis, while extensive, started to heal with diligent care. We continued to monitor his coagulation levels closely, adjusting his warfarin dosage to maintain an optimal balance between preventing new clots and avoiding excessive bleeding.

Finally, after several months of intensive treatment and rehabilitation, the patient was discharged from the hospital. He left with a prescription for oral anticoagulants, a detailed wound care plan, and a schedule for regular follow-up appointments. His leg, while scarred and somewhat weakened, was functional. He had regained his mobility and, more importantly, his appreciation for the importance of proactive healthcare.

CHAPTER TWENTY-ONE
RUN OVER

The shift in the emergency room had been running smoothly until we received the call. An ambulance was en route with a patient who had been run over by his own tractor. Such accidents are not uncommon in rural areas, but they always bring a sense of urgency due to the potential for severe trauma. I braced myself for the worst as the trauma team prepared for the incoming patient.

When the patient arrived, he was in a critical state. He had fallen off his tractor, and the heavy machine had run over his abdomen and lower extremities. The paramedics had already initiated basic life support, and he was intubated due to compromised airway and breathing. His vital signs were unstable: blood pressure was dangerously low at 70/40 mmHg, heart rate was rapid

at 130 beats per minute, and his oxygen saturation was fluctuating around 85%.

The first priority was to stabilize his condition. The patient was immediately placed on a mechanical ventilator to ensure adequate oxygenation. Two large-bore IV lines were established for rapid fluid resuscitation. We administered a bolus of normal saline, followed by a continuous infusion to combat the hypovolemic shock. Despite the fluids, his blood pressure remained critically low, indicating significant internal bleeding. Therefore, we initiated a transfusion of O-negative blood while we awaited the results of his blood type and crossmatch.

A primary survey was conducted to identify life-threatening injuries. The patient's abdomen was distended and tender, with visible bruising and signs of internal bleeding. FAST (Focused Assessment with Sonography for Trauma) ultrasound revealed free fluid in the abdominal cavity, suggesting a hemoperitoneum. The pelvic binder was applied due to suspected pelvic fractures, which are common in such high-energy injuries and can contribute to massive hemorrhage.

The patient was sent for a quick CT scan to get a clearer picture of the extent of his injuries. The CT scan revealed multiple fractures in the pelvis, including an open book fracture, along with significant liver lacerations and splenic injury. His left femur was also frac-

tured, and there was evidence of a potential aortic injury.

Given the severity of the injuries, it was clear that the patient required immediate surgical intervention. We prepared the patient for emergency exploratory laparotomy. The trauma surgeon was on standby as the patient was rushed to the operating room. During the surgery, the surgeon discovered and controlled several sources of bleeding. The liver lacerations were packed, and a splenectomy was performed due to the extent of the splenic injury. The pelvic fractures were stabilized with external fixation. Despite the rapid intervention, the patient continued to require massive transfusions due to ongoing blood loss.

Post-surgery, the patient was transferred to the intensive care unit (ICU) for further management. In the ICU, his condition remained critical. He was placed on vasopressors to maintain his blood pressure and continued to receive blood products. His kidney function was closely monitored due to the risk of acute kidney injury from the shock and massive transfusion. He was also started on broad-spectrum antibiotics to prevent infections, given the splenectomy and open fractures.

The ICU team implemented a comprehensive plan to address the patient's multi-system trauma. This

included ongoing hemodynamic support, ventilator management, and monitoring for complications such as acute respiratory distress syndrome (ARDS) and sepsis. The patient was also started on a pain management regimen, including intravenous opioids and sedatives to ensure comfort and reduce metabolic demand.

Despite the aggressive treatment, the patient's condition remained precarious. Over the next 24 hours, he developed worsening respiratory distress, and repeat chest X-rays showed bilateral infiltrates consistent with ARDS. His renal function also deteriorated, necessitating continuous renal replacement therapy (CRRT) to manage fluid balance and metabolic waste.

Unfortunately, despite all efforts, the patient developed multi-organ failure. His liver function tests worsened, indicating hepatic failure. He became increasingly coagulopathic, and his platelet count dropped despite ongoing transfusions. Despite the best supportive care, he succumbed to his injuries on the third day post-admission.

The patient's death was a sobering reminder of the severe and often insurmountable nature of polytrauma. Reflecting on the case, the emergency team reviewed each step of the management to identify areas for improvement in future cases. The primary and secondary surveys were conducted efficiently, the deci-

sion for rapid surgical intervention was appropriate, and the ICU management followed established protocols. The case underscored the importance of rapid assessment, stabilization, and multidisciplinary care in managing complex trauma patients.

In conclusion, the patient's case was a tragic outcome of a common rural accident. The initial diagnosis included severe blunt abdominal trauma, pelvic fractures, liver and splenic injuries, and potential aortic injury. The treatment plan involved immediate resuscitation, blood transfusion, surgical intervention, and intensive supportive care. Despite the comprehensive and timely medical response, the severity of the injuries led to multi-organ failure and the patient's demise. This case highlights the critical nature of trauma management and the limitations we face despite advanced medical interventions.

CHAPTER TWENTY-TWO
SEVERE PREECLAMPSIA

The night began like any other in the emergency room. The steady hum of activity, the rhythmic beeping of monitors, and the occasional hurried footsteps of the staff set the backdrop for another shift. The doors swung open, and the paramedics wheeled in a patient on a gurney. She was in her third trimester of pregnancy, visibly distressed, and her condition was alarming from the moment I laid eyes on her. Her face was flushed, her breathing rapid, and she clutched her swollen abdomen with one hand while the other gripped the side of the gurney.

The paramedics handed over a brief report: "Severe headache, visual disturbances, and elevated blood pressure," they stated. As I approached the patient, my

immediate concern was preeclampsia, a potentially life-threatening condition for both mother and child. I swiftly directed the team to transfer her to a room and ordered an urgent assessment.

Upon arrival in the room, I conducted a rapid physical examination. Her blood pressure was alarmingly high at 180/120 mmHg. I noted pitting edema in her lower extremities, and she complained of severe upper abdominal pain, a hallmark of preeclampsia. We needed to act quickly to stabilize her condition.

I ordered a series of tests: a complete blood count, liver function tests, kidney function tests, and coagulation profile, along with urine analysis for proteinuria. Simultaneously, I instructed the nurse to start an IV line and administer magnesium sulfate to prevent seizures, a common complication of severe preeclampsia.

While waiting for the lab results, I reviewed the patient's history. She had been experiencing increasing blood pressure over the past few weeks, but it had not been managed effectively. Her prenatal care visits had been sporadic, likely due to socio-economic factors. The lack of consistent monitoring had allowed her condition to escalate unchecked.

The lab results confirmed our suspicions: elevated liver enzymes, thrombocytopenia, and significant

proteinuria. The diagnosis was severe preeclampsia, and the situation was dire. The next step was to control her blood pressure to prevent complications such as eclampsia, stroke, or organ failure.

I prescribed a continuous infusion of labetalol, an antihypertensive medication, to bring her blood pressure under control. The goal was to lower her blood pressure gradually to avoid compromising placental perfusion, which could endanger the fetus. I also ordered betamethasone to promote fetal lung maturity, anticipating a possible premature delivery.

As the medication began to take effect, I monitored the patient's vital signs closely. Her blood pressure showed signs of gradual improvement, but she remained at high risk for complications. I contacted the obstetrics team to prepare for an emergency cesarean section. Delivering the baby was the definitive treatment for preeclampsia, but it required a delicate balance to ensure both mother and child could endure the procedure.

The hours passed in a blur of activity. The patient's condition fluctuated, and she developed signs of pulmonary edema. Her breathing became labored, and her oxygen saturation dropped. I ordered a chest X-ray, which revealed fluid accumulation in her lungs. Imme-

diate intervention was necessary. I adjusted her fluid intake, restricted IV fluids, and administered diuretics to reduce the fluid overload.

Despite these efforts, her condition remained precarious. The obstetrics team arrived, and we discussed the plan. The priority was to stabilize the patient enough to proceed with the delivery. Given her severe preeclampsia and the onset of pulmonary edema, waiting any longer would increase the risk of maternal and fetal mortality.

The decision was made to proceed with an emergency cesarean section. I coordinated with the anesthesiologist to ensure she received the necessary care during surgery. The operating room was prepped, and the patient was wheeled in. The atmosphere was tense, with the lives of two individuals hanging in the balance.

The surgery began, and the obstetrics team worked swiftly and efficiently. The baby was delivered, a premature but otherwise healthy infant, immediately transferred to the neonatal intensive care unit for further care. The focus then shifted entirely to the mother. Her blood pressure remained a concern, and the potential for complications was high.

Post-surgery, the patient was moved to the intensive care unit for close monitoring. The team continued the magnesium sulfate infusion to prevent seizures and

maintained the antihypertensive treatment to manage her blood pressure. I ordered frequent blood tests to monitor her liver and kidney function, as well as her platelet count, to detect any signs of deterioration.

In the ICU, the patient's condition was closely observed. Her blood pressure gradually stabilized, and her respiratory function improved with diuretics and careful fluid management. However, her kidney function remained impaired, suggesting possible acute kidney injury secondary to preeclampsia. I consulted with the nephrology team to manage this complication.

Over the next few days, the patient showed signs of improvement. Her liver enzymes began to normalize, and her platelet count increased. The risk of eclampsia diminished, and we were able to taper off the magnesium sulfate. Her blood pressure, though still elevated, was controlled with oral antihypertensive medications.

The turning point came when her kidney function showed signs of recovery. Urine output increased, and her creatinine levels began to fall. The nephrology team was optimistic about her prognosis, provided she continued to receive appropriate care and follow-up.

By the end of the week, the patient was stable enough to be transferred from the ICU to a regular ward. She remained under close observation, but the immediate life-threatening aspects of her condition had

been managed. The focus shifted to ensuring she received the necessary support for a full recovery and planning her discharge.

The neonatal team reported that the baby, though premature, was doing well. This news provided a much-needed boost to the patient's spirits, which had been understandably low given the ordeal she had endured. We arranged for her to visit the NICU to see her baby, a moment that brought tears to many eyes in the unit.

As the days progressed, the patient continued to improve. Her blood pressure remained stable with oral medications, her kidney function normalized, and her overall condition strengthened. We provided her with detailed instructions for managing her blood pressure at home, emphasizing the importance of regular follow-up visits and adherence to her medication regimen.

Finally, after two weeks of intensive care and monitoring, the patient was discharged. She left the hospital with her baby in her arms, a testament to the resilience and strength of both mother and child. The follow-up plan included regular visits to her obstetrician and primary care physician to monitor her blood pressure and overall health.

In the end, the patient's recovery was a triumph of modern medicine, collaborative care, and her own indomitable will. The sight of her leaving the hospital,

holding her newborn, was a poignant reminder of why we do what we do. The road ahead would still require vigilance and care, but for that moment, we celebrated a hard-fought victory in the face of severe adversity.

———

CONTINUE WITH:

ON CALL: EMERGENCY ROOM STORIES: VOLUME 3

ABOUT THE AUTHOR

Dr. David Berg is a highly skilled and compassionate doctor, specializing in internal medicine. With a passion for patient care, he excels in connecting with individuals on a deep level. Driven by a thirst for knowledge, he has contributed to groundbreaking research and established clinics in underserved communities. His gentle demeanor and commitment to personalized care have made him a beloved figure in the medical community. Dr. David Berg is a beacon of hope, transforming lives and inspiring others to create a healthier world.

He loves humor, his work, as well as his wife and family. He lives north of Houston, in the great state of Texas.

ALSO BY DAVID BERG, M.D.

STAT: CRAZY MEDICAL STORIES

CRASH: STORIES FROM THE EMERGENCY ROOM

ALSO BY FREE REIGN PUBLISHING

ENCOUNTERS IN THE WOODS

WHAT LURKS BEYOND

FEAR IN THE FOREST

INTO THE DARKNESS

ENCOUNTERS BIGFOOT

TALES OF TERROR

I SAW BIGFOOT

STALKED: TERRIFYING TRUE CRIME STORIES

MYSTERIES IN THE DARK

13 PAST MIDNIGHT

THINGS IN THE WOODS

CONSPIRACY THEORIES THAT WERE TRUE

LOVE ENCOUNTERS

STAT: CRAZY MEDICAL STORIES

CRASH: STORIES FROM THE EMERGENCY ROOM

CODE BLUE: TALES FROM THE EMERGENCY ROOM

LEGENDS AND STORIES SERIES

10-33: TRUE TALES FROM THE THIN BLUE LINE

BEYOND THE PATH

FROM ABOVE: UFO ENCOUNTERS

WENDIGO CHRONICLES

MYSTERIES IN THE FOREST

STORIES FROM THE NICU

CRAZY MEDICAL STORIES

PAWSITIVE MOMENTS: LIFE IN A VETERINARY CLINIC

STORIES FROM THE NICU

VANISHED: STRANGE & MYSTERIOUS DISAPPEARANCES

DIAGNOSIS: RARE MEDICAL CASES

THE BIG BIGFOOT BOOK SERIES

THE MEGA MONSTER BOOK SERIES

LOST SOULS: 50 NATIONAL PARK DISAPPEARANCES

ON CALL: EMERGENCY ROOM STORIES

CURSED: TALES OF THE WORLD'S MOST HAUNTED
OBJECTS

CRAZY AMBULANCE STORIES

IN YOUR OWN WORDS GUIDED JOURNAL SERIES

31 A 60/40 portfolio allocation it is a portfolio that holds 60 percent stocks and 40 percent bonds. It is often used as a benchmark for a "balanced" asset allocation.

32 Vernon, Steve. "Planning your retirement: 10 ways to reduce housing costs." Money Watch, 6 May 2013. CBS News. 2014. CBS Interactive Inc.

33 According to the American Bar Association, probate is the formal legal process that gives recognition to a will and appoints the executor or personal representative who will administer the estate and distribute assets to the intended beneficiaries.